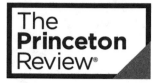

MCAT®

Organic Chemistry Review

3rd Edition

The Staff of The Princeton Review

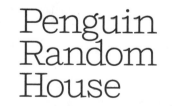

Penguin
Random
House

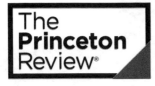

The Princeton Review
24 Prime Parkway, Suite 201
Natick, MA 01760
E-mail: editorialsupport@review.com

Published in the United States by Penguin Random
House LLC, New York, and in Canada by Random House
of Canada, a division of Penguin Random House Ltd.,
Toronto.

The Princeton Review is not affiliated with Princeton
University.

MCAT is a registered trademark of the Association of
American Medical Colleges, which is not affiliated with
The Princeton Review.

ISBN 978-1-101-92058-9
ISSN 2150-8887

Editor: Selena Coppock
Production Editor: Harmony Quiroz
Production Artist: Craig Patches

Printed in the United States of America on partially
recycled paper.

10 9 8 7 6 5 4 3

3rd Edition

Editorial

Rob Franek, Senior VP, Publisher
Casey Cornelius, VP Content Development
Mary Beth Garrick, Director of Production
Selena Coppock, Managing Editor
Meave Shelton, Senior Editor
Colleen Day, Editor
Sarah Litt, Editor
Aaron Riccio, Editor
Orion McBean, Editorial Assistant

Random House Publishing Team

Tom Russell, Publisher
Alison Stoltzfus, Publishing Manager
Melinda Ackell, Associate Managing Editor
Ellen Reed, Production Manager
Kristin Lindner, Production Supervisor
Andrea Lau, Designer

CONTRIBUTORS

Peter J. Alaimo, Ph.D.
        Senior Author

TPR MCAT O-Chem Development Team:

Bethany Blackwell, M.S., Senior Editor

William Ewing, Ph.D.

Brandon Kelley, Ph.D.

Jason Osman, Ph.D., Lead Developer

Edited for Production by:

Judene Wright, M.S., M.A.Ed.
        National Content Director, MCAT Program, The Princeton Review

The TPR MCAT O-Chem Team and Judene would like to thank the following people for their contributions to this book:

Farhad Aziz, B.S., Kristen Brunson, Ph.D., Brian Butts, B.S., B.A., Douglas S. Daniels, Ph.D., Amanda Edward, H.BSc, H.BEd, Carlos Guzman, Adam Johnson, Omair Adil Khan, Stefan Loren, Ph.D., Joey Mancuso, D.O., M.S., Janet Marshall, Ph.D., Douglas K. McLemore, B.S., Katherine Miller, B.A., Tenaya Newkirk, Ph.D., Daniel J. Pallin, M.D., Tyler Peikes, Chris Rabbat, Ph.D., Steven Rines, Ph.D., Jayson Sack, M.D., M.S., Karen Salazar, Ph.D., Sina Shahbaz, B.S., Christopher Volpe, Ph.D.

Periodic Table of the Elements

1 H 1.0																	2 He 4.0
3 Li 6.9	4 Be 9.0											5 B 10.8	6 C 12.0	7 N 14.0	8 O 16.0	9 F 19.0	10 Ne 20.2
11 Na 23.0	12 Mg 24.3											13 Al 27.0	14 Si 28.1	15 P 31.0	16 S 32.1	17 Cl 35.5	18 Ar 39.9
19 K 39.1	20 Ca 40.1	21 Sc 45.0	22 Ti 47.9	23 V 50.9	24 Cr 52.0	25 Mn 54.9	26 Fe 55.8	27 Co 58.9	28 Ni 58.7	29 Cu 63.5	30 Zn 65.4	31 Ga 69.7	32 Ge 72.6	33 As 74.9	34 Se 79.0	35 Br 79.9	36 Kr 83.8
37 Rb 85.5	38 Sr 87.6	39 Y 88.9	40 Zr 91.2	41 Nb 92.9	42 Mo 95.9	43 Tc (98)	44 Ru 101.1	45 Rh 102.9	46 Pd 106.4	47 Ag 107.9	48 Cd 112.4	49 In 114.8	50 Sn 118.7	51 Sb 121.8	52 Te 127.6	53 I 126.9	54 Xe 131.3
55 Cs 132.9	56 Ba 137.3	57 *La 138.9	72 Hf 178.5	73 Ta 180.9	74 W 183.9	75 Re 186.2	76 Os 190.2	77 Ir 192.2	78 Pt 195.1	79 Au 197.0	80 Hg 200.6	81 Tl 204.4	82 Pb 207.2	83 Bi 209.0	84 Po (209)	85 At (210)	86 Rn (222)
87 Fr (223)	88 Ra 226.0	89 †Ac 227.0	104 Rf (261)	105 Db (262)	106 Sg (266)	107 Bh (264)	108 Hs (277)	109 Mt (268)	110 Ds (281)	111 Rg (272)	112 Cn (285)	113 Uut (286)	114 Fl (289)	115 Uup (288)	116 Lv (293)	117 Uus (294)	118 Uuo (294)

*Lanthanide Series:

58 Ce 140.1	59 Pr 140.9	60 Nd 144.2	61 Pm (145)	62 Sm 150.4	63 Eu 152.0	64 Gd 157.3	65 Tb 158.9	66 Dy 162.5	67 Ho 164.9	68 Er 167.3	69 Tm 168.9	70 Yb 173.0	71 Lu 175.0

†Actinide Series:

90 Th 232.0	91 Pa (231)	92 U 238.0	93 Np (237)	94 Pu (244)	95 Am (243)	96 Cm (247)	97 Bk (247)	98 Cf (251)	99 Es (252)	100 Fm (257)	101 Md (258)	102 No (259)	103 Lr (260)

MCAT ORGANIC CHEMISTRY REVIEW CONTENTS

Register Your

1 Go to **PrincetonReview.com/cracking**

2 You'll see a welcome page where you should register your book or boxed set of books using the ISBN. If you have a book, the ISBN can be found above the bar code on the back cover. If you have a boxed set, the ISBN can be found on the back of the box above the bar code.

3 After placing this free order, you'll either be asked to log in or to answer a few simple questions in order to set up a new Princeton Review account.

4 Finally, click on the "Student Tools" tab located at the top of the screen. It may take an hour or two for your registration to go through, but after that, you're good to go.

NOTE: If you are experiencing book problems (potential content errors), please contact EditorialSupport@review.com with the full title of the book, its ISBN number, and the page number of the error.

Experiencing technical issues? Please email TPRStudentTech@review.com with the following information:

- your full name
- e-mail address used to register the book
- full book title and ISBN
- your computer OS (Mac or PC) and Internet browser (Firefox, Safari, Chrome, etc.)
- description of technical issue

Book Online!

Once you've registered, you can...

· Take 3 full-length practice MCAT exams
· Find useful information about taking the MCAT and applying to medical school
· Check to see if there have been any updates to this edition

Offline Resources

If you are looking for more review or medical school advice, please feel free to pick up these books in stores right now!

· *Medical School Essays That Made a Difference*
· *The Best 167 Medical Schools*
· *The Princeton Review Complete MCAT*

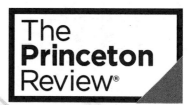

Chapter 1
MCAT Basics

SO YOU WANT TO BE A DOCTOR

So...you want to be a doctor. If you're like most premeds, you've wanted to be a doctor since you were pretty young. When people asked you what you wanted to be when you grew up, you always answered "a doctor." You had toy medical kits, bandaged up your dog or cat, and played "hospital." You probably read your parents' home medical guides for fun.

When you got to high school you took the honors and AP classes. You studied hard, got straight As (or, at least, really good grades!), and participated in extracurricular activities so you could get into a good college. And you succeeded!

At college you knew exactly what to do. You took your classes seriously, studied hard, and got a great GPA. You talked to your professors and hung out at office hours to get good letters of recommendation. You were a member of the premed society on campus, volunteered at hospitals, and shadowed doctors. All that's left to do now is to get a good MCAT score.

Just the MCAT.

Just the most confidence-shattering, most demoralizing, longest, most brutal entrance exam for any graduate program. At about 7.5 hours (including breaks), the MCAT tops the list; even the closest runners up, the LSAT and GMAT, are only about 4 hours long. The MCAT tests significant science content knowledge along with the ability to think quickly, reason logically, and read comprehensively, all under the pressure of a timed exam.

The path to a good MCAT score is not as easy to see as the path to a good GPA or the path to a good letter of recommendation. The MCAT is less about what you know and more about how to apply what you know—and how to apply it quickly to new situations. Because the path might not be so clear, you might be worried. That's why you picked up this book.

We promise to demystify the MCAT for you, with clear descriptions of the different sections, how the test is scored, and what the test experience is like. We will help you understand general test-taking techniques as well as provide you with specific techniques for each section. We will review the science content you need to know as well as give you strategies for the Organic Chemistry section. We'll show you the path to a good MCAT score and help you walk the path.

After all, you want to be a doctor. And we want you to succeed.

WHAT IS THE MCAT...REALLY?

Most test-takers approach the MCAT as though it were a typical college science test, one in which facts and knowledge simply need to be regurgitated in order to do well. They study for the MCAT the same way they did for their college tests, by memorizing facts and details, formulas and equations. And when they get to the MCAT they are surprised...and disappointed.

It's a myth that the MCAT is purely a content-knowledge test. If medical school admission committees want to see what you know, all they have to do is look at your transcripts. What they really want to see is how you think, especially under pressure. That's what your MCAT score will tell them.

The MCAT is really a test of your ability to apply basic knowledge to different, possibly new, situations. It's a test of your ability to reason out and evaluate arguments. Do you still need to know your science content? Absolutely. But not at the level that most test-takers think they need to know it. Furthermore, your science knowledge won't help you on the Critical Analysis and Reasoning Skills (CARS) section. So how do you study for a test like this?

You study for the science sections by reviewing the basics and then applying them to MCAT practice questions. You study for the CARS section by learning how to adapt your existing reading and analytical skills to the nature of the test (more information about the CARS section can be found in *MCAT Critical Analysis and Reasoning Skills Review*).

The book you are holding will review all the relevant MCAT Organic Chemistry content you will need for the test, and a little bit more. It includes hundreds of questions (printed and online) designed to make you think about the material in a deeper way, along with full explanations to clarify the logical thought process needed to get to the answer. It also comes with access to three full-length online practice exams to further hone your skills. For more information on accessing those online exams, please refer to the "Register Your Book Online!" spread on page viii.

A Note About Flashcards

For most of the exams you've taken previously, flashcards were likely very helpful. This was because those exams mostly required you to regurgitate information, and flashcards are pretty good at helping you memorize facts. However, the most challenging aspect of the MCAT is not that it requires you to memorize the fine details of content knowledge, but that it requires you to apply your basic scientific knowledge to unfamiliar situations: flashcards alone may not help you there.

Flashcards can be beneficial if your basic content knowledge is deficient in some area. For example, if you don't know the definitions of all the possible types of isomers, or if you are unsure of some of the functional groups you need to know, flashcards can certainly help you memorize these facts. Or, you may need to learn and recognize polar, nonpolar, acidic, and basic amino acids and their 1-letter abbreviations. You might find that flashcards can help you memorize these. But unless you are trying to memorize basic facts in your personal weak areas, you are better off doing and analyzing practice passages than carrying around a stack of flashcards.

MCAT NUTS AND BOLTS

Overview

The MCAT is a computer-based test (CBT) that is *not* adaptive. Adaptive tests base your next question on whether or not you've answered the current question correctly. The MCAT is linear, or fixed-form, meaning that the questions are in a predetermined order and do not change based on your answers. However, there are many versions of the test so that on a given test day, different people will see different versions. The following table highlights the features of the MCAT exam.

Registration	Online via www.aamc.org. Begins as early as six months prior to test date; available up until week of test (subject to seat availability).
Testing Centers	Administered at small, secure, climate-controlled computer testing rooms.
Security	Photo ID with signature, electronic fingerprint, electronic signature verification, assigned seat
Proctoring	None. Test administrator checks examinee in and assigns seat at computer. All testing instructions are given on the computer.
Frequency of Test	Many times per year distributed over January, April, May, June, July, August, and September.
Format	Exclusively computer-based. NOT an adaptive test.
Length of Test Day	7.5 hours.
Breaks	Optional 10-minute breaks between sections, with a 30-minute break for lunch.
Section Names	1. Chemical and Physical Foundations of Biological Systems (Chem/Phys) 2. Critical Analysis and Reasoning Skills (CARS) 3. Biological and Biochemical Foundations of Living Systems (Bio/Biochem) 4. Psychological, Social, and Biological Foundations of Behavior (Psych/Soc)
Number of Questions and Timing	59 Chem/Phys questions, 95 minutes 53 CARS questions, 90 minutes 59 Bio/Biochem questions, 95 minutes 59 Psych/Soc questions, 95 minutes
Scoring	Test is scaled. Several forms per administration.
Allowed/Not allowed	No timers/watches. Noise reduction headphones available. Unopened package of foam earplugs is allowed. Scratch paper and pencils given at start of test and taken at end of test. Locker or secure area provided for personal items.
Results: Timing and Delivery	Approximately 30 days. Electronic scores only, available online through AAMC login. Examinees can print official score reports.
Maximum Number of Retakes	As of April 2015, the MCAT can be taken a maximum of three times in one year, four times over two years, and seven times over the lifetime of the examinee. An examinee can only be registered for one date at a time.

Registration

Registration for the exam is completed online at https://www.aamc.org/students/applying/mcat/reserving. The AAMC opens registration for a given test date at least two months in advance of the date, often earlier. It's a good idea to register well in advance of your desired test date to make sure that you get a seat.

Sections

There are four sections on the MCAT exam: Chemical and Physical Foundations of Biological Systems (Chem/Phys), Critical Analysis and Reasoning Skills (CARS), Biological and Biochemical Foundations of Living Systems (Bio/Biochem), and Psychological, Social, and Biological Foundations of Behavior (Psych/Soc). All sections consist of multiple-choice questions.

Section	Concepts Tested	Number of Questions and Timing
Chemical and Physical Foundations of Biological Systems	Basic concepts in chemistry and physics, including biochemistry, scientific inquiry, reasoning, research methods, and statistics.	59 questions, 95 minutes
Critical Analysis and Reasoning Skills	Critical analysis of information drawn from a wide range of social science and humanities disciplines.	53 questions, 90 minutes
Biological and Biochemical Foundations of Living Systems	Basic concepts in biology and biochemistry, scientific inquiry, reasoning, research methods, and statistics.	59 questions, 95 minutes
Psychological, Social, and Biological Foundations of Behavior	Basic concepts in psychology, sociology, and biology, scientific inquiry, reasoning, research methods, and statistics.	59 questions, 95 minutes

Most questions on the MCAT (44 in the science sections, all 53 in the CARS section) are **passage-based**; the science sections have 10 passages each and the CARS section has 9. A passage consists of a few paragraphs of information on which several following questions are based. In the science sections, passages often include equations or reactions, tables, graphs, figures, and experiments to analyze. CARS passages come from literature in the social sciences, humanities, ethics, philosophy, cultural studies, and population health, and do not test content knowledge in any way.

Some questions in the science sections are **freestanding questions (FSQs)**. These questions are independent of any passage information and appear in several groups of about four to five questions, interspersed throughout the passages. 15 of the questions in the science sections are freestanding, and the remainder are passage-based.

Each section on the MCAT is separated by either a 10-minute break or a 30-minute lunch break.

Section	Time
Test Center Check-In	Variable, can take up to 40 minutes if center is busy.
Tutorial	10 minutes
Chemical and Physical Foundations of Biological Systems	95 minutes
Break	10 minutes
Critical Analysis and Reasoning Skills	90 minutes
Lunch Break	30 minutes
Biological and Biochemical Foundations of Living Systems	95 minutes
Break	10 minutes
Psychological, Social, and Biological Foundations of Behavior	95 minutes
Void Option	5 minutes
Survey	5 minutes

The survey includes questions about your satisfaction with the overall MCAT experience, including registration, check-in, etc., as well as questions about how you prepared for the test.

Scoring

The MCAT is a scaled exam, meaning that your raw score will be converted into a scaled score that takes into account the difficulty of the questions. There is no guessing penalty. All sections are scored from 118–132, with a total scaled score range of 472–528. Because different versions of the test have varying levels of difficulty, the scale will be different from one exam to the next. Thus, there is no "magic number" of questions to get right in order to get a particular score. Plus, some of the questions on the test are considered "experimental" and do not count toward your score; they are just there to be evaluated for possible future inclusion in a test.

At the end of the test (after you complete the Psychological, Social, and Biological Foundations of Behavior section), you will be asked to choose one of the following two options: "I wish to have my MCAT exam scored" or "I wish to VOID my MCAT exam." You have five minutes to make a decision, and if you do not select one of the options in that time, the test will automatically be scored. If you choose the VOID option, your test will not be scored (you will not now, or ever, get a numerical score for this test), medical schools will not know you took the test, and no refunds will be granted. You cannot "unvoid" your scores at a later time.

So, what's a good score? The AAMC is centering the scale at 500 (i.e., 500 will be the 50th percentile), and recommends that application committees consider applicants near the center of the range. To be on the safe side, aim for a total score of around 510. Remember that if your GPA is on the low side, you'll need higher MCAT scores to compensate, and if you have a strong GPA, you can get away with lower MCAT scores. But the reality is that your chances of acceptance depend on a lot more than just your MCAT scores. It's a combination of your GPA, your MCAT scores, your undergraduate coursework, letters of recommendation, experience related to the medical field (such as volunteer work or research), extracurricular activities, your personal statement, etc. Medical schools are looking for a complete package, not just good scores and a good GPA.

GENERAL LAYOUT AND TEST-TAKING STRATEGIES

Layout of the Test

In each section of the test, the computer screen is divided vertically, with the passage on the left and the range of questions for that passage indicated above (e.g. "Passage 1 Questions 1–5"). The scroll bar for the passage text appears in the middle of the screen. Each question appears on the right, and you need to click "Next" to move to each subsequent question.

In the science sections, the freestanding questions are found in groups of 4–5, interspersed with the passages. The screen is still divided vertically; on the left is the statement "Questions [X–XX] do not refer to a passage and are independent of each other" and each question appears on the right as described above.

CBT Tools

There are a number of tools available on the test, including highlighting, strike-outs, the Mark button, the Review button, the Periodic Table button, and of course, scratch paper. The following is a brief description of each tool.

1) **Highlighting:** This is done in the passage text (including table entries and some equations, but excluding figures and molecular structures) and in the question stems by left-clicking and dragging the mouse across the words you wish to highlight; the selected words will then be highlighted in blue. When you release the mouse, a highlighting icon will appear; clicking on the icon will highlight the selected text in yellow. To remove the highlighting, left-click on the highlighted text.

2) **Strike-outs:** Right-clicking on an answer choice causes the entire text of that choice to be crossed out. The strike-out can be removed by right-clicking again. Left-clicking selects an answer choice; note than an answer choice that is selected cannot be struck out. When you strike out a figure or molecular structure, instead of being crossed out, the image turns grey.

3) **Mark button:** This allows you to flag the question for later review. When clicked, the flag on the "Mark" button turns red and says "Marked."

4) **Review button:** Clicking this button brings up a new screen showing all questions and their status (either "completed," "incomplete," or "marked"). You can choose to: "review all," "review incomplete," or "review marked." You can also double-click any question number to quickly return to that specific question. You can only review questions in the section of the MCAT you are currently taking, but the Review button can be clicked at any time during the allotted time for that section; you do NOT have to wait until the end of the section to click it.

5) **Periodic Table button:** Clicking this button will open a periodic table. Note that the periodic table is large, however it can be resized to see the questions and a portion of the periodic table at the same time.

6) **Scratch paper:** You will be given four pages (8 faces) of scratch paper at the start of the test. You can ask for more at any point during the test, and your first set of paper will be collected before you receive fresh paper. Scratch paper is only useful if it is kept organized; do not give in to the tendency to write on the first available open space! Good organization will be very helpful when/if you wish to review a question. Indicate the passage number and the range of questions for that passage in a box near the top of your scratch work, and indicate the question you are working on in a circle to the left of the notes for that question. Draw a line under your scratch work when you change passages to keep the work separate. Do not erase or scribble over any previous work. If you do not think it is correct, draw one line through the work and start again. You may have already done some useful work without realizing it.

General Strategy for the Science Sections

Passages vs. FSQs in the Science Sections: What to Start With

Since the questions are displayed on separate screens, it is awkward and time consuming to click through all of the questions up front to find the FSQs. Therefore, go through the section on a first pass and decide whether to do the passage now or to save it for later, basing your decision on the passage text and the first question. Tackle the FSQs as you come upon them. More details are below.

Here is an outline of the procedure:

1) For each passage, write a heading on your scratch paper with the passage number, the general topic, and its range of questions (e.g. "Passage 1, thermodynamics, Q 1–5" or "Passage 2, enzymes, Q 6–9). The passage numbers do not currently appear in the Review screen, thus having the question numbers on your scratch paper will allow you to move through the section more efficiently.
2) Skim the text and rank the passage. If a passage is a "Now," complete it before moving on to the next passage (also see "Attacking the Questions" below). If it is a "Later" passage, first write "SKIPPED" in block letters under the passage heading on your scratch paper and leave room for your work when you come back to complete that passage. (Note that the specific passages you skip will be unique to you; in the Bio/Biochem section, you might choose to do all Biology passages first, then come back for Biochemistry. Or in Chem/Phys you might choose to skip experiment-based or analytical passages. Know ahead of time what type of passage you are going to skip and follow your plan.)
3) Next, click on the "Review" button at the bottom to get to the review screen. Double-click on the first question of the next passage; you'll be able to identify it because you know the range of questions from the passage you just skipped. This will take you to the next passage, where you will repeat steps 1–3.
4) Once you have completed the "Now" passages, go to the review screen and double-click the first question for the first passage you skipped. Answer the questions, and continue going back to the review screen and repeating this procedure for other passages you have skipped.

Attacking the Questions

As you work through the questions, if you encounter a particularly lengthy question, or a question that requires a lot of analysis, you may choose to skip it. This is a wise strategy because it ensures you will tackle all the easier questions first, the ones you are more likely to get right. If you choose to skip the question, (or if you attempt it but get stuck), write down the question number on your scratch paper, click the Mark button to flag the question in the Review screen, and move on to the next question. At the end of the passage, click back through the set of questions to complete any that you skipped over the first time through, and make sure that you have filled in an answer for every question.

General Strategy for the CARS Section

Ranking and Ordering the Passages: What to Start With

Ranking: Since the questions are displayed on separate screens, it is awkward and time consuming to click through all of the questions before ranking each passage as Now (an easier passage), Later (a harder passage), or Killer (a passage that you will randomly guess on). Therefore, rank the passage and decide whether or not to do it on the first pass through the section based on the passage text, skimming the first 2–3 sentences.

Ordering: Because of the additional clicking through screens (or, use of the Review screen) that is required to navigate through the section, the "Two-Pass" system (completing the "Now" passages as you find them) is likely to be your most efficient approach. However, if you find that you are continuously making a lot of bad ranking decisions, it is still valid to experiment with the "Three-Pass" approach (ranking all nine passages up front before attempting your first "Now" passage).

Here is an outline of the basic Ranking and Ordering procedure to follow.

1) For each passage, write a heading on your scratch paper with the passage number and its range of questions (e.g. "Passage 1 Q 1–7). The passage numbers do not currently appear in the Review screen, thus having the question numbers on your scratch paper will allow you to move through the section more efficiently.

2) Skim the first 2–3 sentences and rank the passage. If the passage is a "Now," complete it before moving on to the next. If it is a "Later" or "Killer," first write either "Later" or "Killer" and "SKIPPED" in block letters under the passage heading on your scratch paper and leave room for your work if you decide to come back and complete that passage. Then click through each question, marking each one and filling in random guesses, until you get to the next passage.

3) Once you have completed the "Now" passages, come back for your second pass and complete the "Later" passages, leaving your random guesses in place for any "Killer" passages that you choose not to complete. Go to the Review screen and use your scratch paper notes on the question numbers; double-click on the number of the first question for that passage to go back to that question, and proceed from there. Alternatively, if you have consistently marked all the questions for passages you skipped in your first pass you can use "Review Marked" from the Review screen to find and complete your "Later" passages.

4) Regardless of how you choose to find your second pass passages, unmark each question after you complete it, so that you can continue to rely on the Review screen (and the "Review Marked" function") to identify questions that you have not yet attempted.

Previewing the Questions

The formatting and functioning of the tools facilitates effective previewing. Having each question on a separate screen will encourage you to really focus on that question. Even more importantly, you can now highlight in the question stem (but still not in the answer choices).

Here is the basic procedure for previewing the questions:

1) Start with the first question, and if it has lead words referencing passage content, highlight them. You may also choose to jot them down on your scratch paper. Once you reach and preview the last question for the set on that passage, THEN stay on that screen and work the passage (your highlighting appears and stays on every passage screen, and persists through the whole 90 minutes).

2) Once you have worked the passage and defined the Bottom Line—the main idea and tone of the entire passage—work backward from the last question to the first. If you skip over any questions as you go (see "Attacking the Questions" below), write down the question number on your scratch paper. Then click **forward** through the set of questions, completing any that you skipped over the first time through. Once you reach and complete the last question for that passage, clicking "Next" will send you to the first question of the next passage. Working the questions from last to first the first time through the set will eliminate the need to click back through multiple screens to get to the first question immediately after previewing, and will also make it easier and more efficient to do the hardest questions last (see "Attacking the Questions" on the next page).

Attacking the Questions

The question types and the procedure for actually attacking each type will be discussed later. However, it is still important **not** to attempt the hardest questions first (potentially getting stuck, wasting time, and discouraging yourself).

So, as you work the questions from last to first (see "Previewing the Questions" above), if you encounter a particularly difficult and/or lengthy question (or if you attempt a question but get stuck) write down the question number on your scratch paper (you may also choose to mark it) and move on backward to the next question. Then click **forward** through the set and complete any that you skipped over the first time through the set, unmarking any questions that you marked that first time through and making sure that you have filled in an answer for every question.

Pacing Strategy for the MCAT

Since the MCAT is a timed test, you must keep an eye on the timer and adjust your pacing as necessary. It would be terrible to run out of time at the end only to discover that the last few questions could have been easily answered in just a few seconds each.

In the science sections you will have about one minute and thirty-five seconds (1:35) per question, and in the CARS section you will have about one minute and forty seconds (1:40) per question (not taking into account time reading the passage before answering the questions).

Section	# of Questions in passage	Approximate time (including reading the passage)
Chem/Phys, Bio/Biochem, and Psych/Soc	4	6.5 minutes
	5	8 minutes
	6	9.5 minutes
CARS	5	8.5 minutes
	6	10 minutes
	7	11.5 minutes

When starting a passage in the science sections, make note of how much time you will allot for it, and the starting time on the timer. Jot down on your scratch paper what the timer should say at the end of the passage. Then just keep an eye on it as you work through the questions. If you are near the end of the time for that passage, guess on any remaining questions, make some notes on your scratch paper, Mark the questions, and move on. Come back to those questions if you have time.

For the CARS section, keep in mind is that many people will maximize their score by *not* trying to complete every question or every passage in the section. A good strategy for test takers who cannot achieve a high level of accuracy on all nine passages is to randomly guess on at least one passage in the section, and spend your time getting a high percentage of the other questions right. To complete all nine CARS passages, you have about ten minutes per passage. To complete eight of the nine, you have about 11 minutes per passage.

To help maximize your number of correct answer choices in any section, do the questions and passages within that section in the order *you* want to do them in. See "General Strategy" above.

Process of Elimination

Process of elimination (POE) is probably the most useful technique you have to tackle MCAT questions. Since there is no guessing penalty, POE allows you to increase your probability of choosing the correct answer by eliminating those you are sure are wrong.

1) Strike out any choices that you are sure are incorrect or that do not address the issue raised in the question.

2) Jot down some notes to help clarify your thoughts if you return to the question.

3) Use the "Mark" button to flag the question for review. (Note, however, that in the CARS section, you generally should not be returning to rethink questions once you have moved on to a new passage.)

4) Do not leave it blank! For the sciences, if you are not sure and you have already spent more than 60 seconds on that question, just pick one of the remaining choices. If you have time to review it at the end, you can always debate the remaining choices based on your previous notes. For CARS, if you have been through the choices two or three times, have re-read the question stem and gone back to the passage, and you are still stuck, move on. Do the remaining questions for that passage, take one more look at the question you were stuck on, then pick an answer and move on for good.

5) Special Note: if three of the four answer choices have been eliminated, the remaining choice must be the correct answer. Don't waste time pondering *why* it is correct, just click it and move on. The MCAT doesn't care if you truly understand why it's the right answer, only that you have the right answer selected.

6) More subject-specific information on techniques will be presented in the next chapter.

Guessing

Remember, there is NO guessing penalty on the MCAT. NEVER leave a question blank!

QUESTION TYPES

In the science sections of the MCAT, the questions fall into one of three main categories.

1) Memory questions: These questions can be answered directly from prior knowledge and represent about 25 percent of the total number of questions.

2) Explicit questions: These questions are those for which the answer is explicitly stated in the passage. To answer them correctly, for example, may just require finding a definition, or reading a graph, or making a simple connection. Explicit questions represent about 35 percent of the total number of questions.

3) Implicit questions: These questions require you to apply knowledge to a new situation; the answer is typically implied by the information in the passage. These questions often start "if.... then...." (for example, "if we modify the experiment in the passage like this, then what result would we expect?"). Implicit style questions make up about 40 percent of the total number of questions.

In the CARS section, the questions fall into four main categories:

1) Specific questions: These either ask you for facts from the passage (Retrieval questions) or require you to deduce what is most likely to be true based on the passage (Inference questions).

2) General questions: These ask you to summarize themes (Main Idea and Primary Purpose questions) or evaluate an author's opinion (Tone/Attitude questions).

3) Reasoning questions: These ask you to describe the purpose of, or the support provided for, a statement made in the passage (Structure questions) or to judge how well the author supports his or her argument (Evaluate questions).

4) Application questions: These ask you to apply new information from either the question stem itself (New Information questions) or from the answer choices (Strengthen, Weaken, and Analogy questions) to the passage.

More detail on question types and strategies can be found in Chapter 2.

TESTING TIPS

Before Test Day

- Take a trip to the test center at least a day or two before your actual test date so that you can easily find the building and room on test day. This will also allow you to gauge traffic and see if you need money for parking or anything like that. Knowing this type of information ahead of time will greatly reduce your stress on the day of your test.
- During the week before the test, adjust your sleeping schedule so that you are going to bed and getting up in the morning at the same times as on the day before and morning of the MCAT. Prioritize getting a reasonable amount of sleep during the last few nights before the test.
- Don't do any heavy studying the day before the test. This is not a test you can cram for! Your goal at this point is to rest and relax so that you can go into test day in a good physical and mental condition.
- Eat well. Try to avoid excessive caffeine and sugar. Ideally, in the weeks leading up to the actual test you should experiment a little bit with foods and practice tests to see which foods give you the most endurance. Aim for steady blood sugar levels during the test: sports drinks, peanut-butter crackers, trail mix, etc. make good snacks for your breaks and lunch.

General Test Day Info and Tips

- On the day of the test, arrive at the test center at least a half hour prior to the start time of your test.
- Examinees will be checked in to the center in the order in which they arrive.
- You will be assigned a locker or secure area in which to put your personal items. Textbooks and study notes are not allowed, so there is no need to bring them with you to the test center.
- Your ID will be checked, a digital image of your fingerprint will be taken, and you will be asked to sign in.
- You will be given scratch paper and a couple of pencils, and the test center administrator will take you to the computer on which you will complete the test. You may not choose a computer; you must use the computer assigned to you.
- Nothing, not even your watch, is allowed at the computer station except your photo ID, your locker key (if provided), and a factory sealed packet of ear plugs.
- If you choose to leave the testing room at the breaks, you will have your fingerprint checked again, and you will have to sign in and out.
- You are allowed to access the items in your locker, except for notes and cell phones. (Check your test center's policy on cell phones ahead of time; some centers do not even allow them to be kept in your locker.)
- Don't forget to bring the snack foods and lunch you experimented with in your practice tests.
- At the end of the test, the test administrator will collect your scratch paper and shred it.
- Definitely take the breaks! Get up and walk around. It's a good way to clear your head between sections and get the blood (and oxygen!) flowing to your brain.
- Ask for new scratch paper at the breaks if you use it all up.

Chapter 2
Organic Chemistry
Strategy for the MCAT

2.1 GENERAL SCIENCE SECTIONS OVERVIEW

There are three science sections on the MCAT:

- Chemical and Physical Foundations of Biological Systems
- Biological and Biochemical Foundations of Living Systems
- Psychological, Social, and Biological Foundations of Behavior

The Chemical and Physical Foundations of Biological Systems section (Chem/Phys) is the first section on the test. It includes questions from General Chemistry (about 35%), Physics (about 25%), Organic Chemistry (about 15%), and Biochemistry (about 25%). Further, the questions often test chemical and physical concepts within a biological setting, for example, pressure and fluid flow in blood vessels. A solid grasp of math fundamentals is required (arithmetic, algebra, graphs, trigonometry, vectors, proportions, and logarithms), however there are no calculus-based questions.

The Biological and Biochemical Foundations of Living Systems section (Bio/Biochem) is the third section on the test. Approximately 65% of the questions in this section come from biology, approximately 25% come from biochemistry, and approximately 10% come from Organic and General Chemistry. Math calculations are generally not required on this section of the test, however a basic understanding of statistics as used in biological research is helpful.

The Psychological, Social, and Biological Foundations of Behavior section (Psych/Soc) is the fourth and final section on the test. About 60% of the questions will be drawn from Psychology, about 30% from Sociology, and about 10% from Biology. As with the Bio/Biochem section, calculations are generally not required, however a basic understanding of statistics as used in research is helpful.

Most of the questions in the science sections (44 of the 59) are passage-based, and each section has ten passages. Passages consist of a few paragraphs of information and include equations, reactions, graphs, figures, tables, experiments, and data. Four to six questions will be associated with each passage.

The remaining 25% of the questions (15 of 59) in each science section are freestanding questions (FSQs). These questions appear in approximately four groups interspersed between the passages. Each group contains four to five questions.

95 minutes are allotted to each of the science sections. This breaks down to approximately one minute and 35 seconds per question.

2.2   GENERAL SCIENCE PASSAGE TYPES

The passages in the science sections fall into one of three main categories: Information and/or Situation Presentation, Experiment/Research Presentation, or Persuasive Reasoning.

Information and/or Situation Presentation

These passages either present straightforward scientific information or they describe a particular event or occurrence. Generally, questions associated with these passages test basic science facts or ask you to predict outcomes given new variables or new information. Here is an example of an Information/Situation Presentation passage:

Figure 1 shows a portion of the inner mechanism of a typical home smoke detector. It consists of a pair of capacitor plates which are charged by a 9-volt battery (not shown). The capacitor plates (electrodes) are connected to a sensor device, D; the resistor R denotes the internal resistance of the sensor. Normally, air acts as an insulator and no current would flow in the circuit shown. However, inside the smoke detector is a small sample of an artificially produced radioactive element, americium-241, which decays primarily by emitting alpha particles, with a half-life of approximately 430 years. The daughter nucleus of the decay has a half-life in excess of two million years and therefore poses virtually no biohazard.

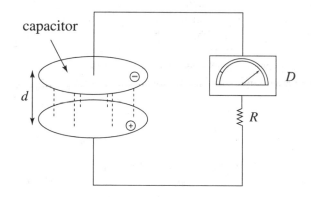

Figure 1   Smoke detector mechanism

The decay products (alpha particles and gamma rays) from the ^{241}Am sample ionize air molecules between the plates and thus provide a conducting pathway which allows current to flow in the circuit shown in Figure 1. A steady-state current is quickly established and remains as long as the battery continues to maintain a 9-volt potential difference between its terminals. However, if smoke particles enter the space between the capacitor plates and thereby interrupt the flow, the current is reduced, and the sensor responds to this change by triggering the alarm. (Furthermore, as the battery starts to "die out," the resulting drop in current is also detected to alert the homeowner to replace the battery.)

$$C = \varepsilon_0 \frac{A}{d}$$

Equation 1

where ε_0 is the universal permittivity constant, equal to 8.85 $\times 10^{-12}$ C^2/(N·m^2). Since the area A of each capacitor plate in the smoke detector is 20 cm^2 and the plates are separated by a distance d of 5 mm, the capacitance is 3.5×10^{-12} F = 3.5 pF.

Experiment/Research Presentation

These passages present the details of experiments and research procedures. They often include data tables and graphs. Generally, questions associated with these passages ask you to interpret data, draw conclusions, and make inferences. Here is an example of an Experiment/Research Presentation passage:

The development of sexual characteristics depends upon various factors, the most important of which are hormonal control, environmental stimuli, and the genetic makeup of the individual. The hormones that contribute to the development include the steroid hormones estrogen, progesterone, and testosterone, as well as the pituitary hormones FSH (follicle-stimulating hormone) and LH (luteinizing hormone).

To study the mechanism by which estrogen exerts its effects, a researcher performed the following experiments using cell culture assays.

Experiment 1:

Human embryonic placental mesenchyme (HEPM) cells were grown for 48 hours in Dulbecco's Modified Eagle Medium (DMEM), with media change every 12 hours. Upon confluent growth, cells were exposed to a 10 mg per mL solution of green fluorescent-labeled estrogen for 1 hour. Cells were rinsed with DMEM and observed under confocal fluorescent microscopy.

Experiment 2:

HEPM cells were grown to confluence as in Experiment 1. Cells were exposed to Pesticide A for 1 hour, followed by the 10 mg/mL solution of labeled estrogen, rinsed as in Experiment 1, and observed under confocal fluorescent microscopy.

Experiment 3:

Experiment 1 was repeated with Chinese Hamster Ovary (CHO) cells instead of HEPM cells.

Experiment 4:

CHO cells injected with cytoplasmic extracts of HEPM cells were grown to confluence, exposed to the 10 mg/mL solution of labeled estrogen for 1 hour, and observed under confocal fluorescent microscopy.

The results of these experiments are given in Table 1.

Table 1 Detection of Estrogen (+ indicates presence of Estrogen)

Experiment	Media	Cytoplasm	Nucleus
1	+	+	+
2	+	+	+
3	+	+	+
4	+	+	+

After observing the cells in each experiment, the researcher bathed the cells in a solution containing 10 mg per mL of a red fluorescent probe that binds specifically to the estrogen receptor only when its active site is occupied. After 1 hour, the cells were rinsed with DMEM and observed under confocal fluorescent microscopy. The results are presented in Table 2.

The researcher also repeated Experiment 2 using Pesticide B, an estrogen analog, instead of Pesticide A. Results from other researchers had shown that Pesticide B binds to the active site of the cytosolic estrogen receptor (with an affinity 10,000 times greater than that of estrogen) and causes increased transcription of mRNA.

Table 2 Observed Fluorescence and Estrogen Effects (G = green, R = red)

Experiment	Media	Cytoplasm	Nucleus	Estrogen effects observed?
1	G only	G and R	G and R	Yes
2	G only	G only	G only	No
3	G only	G only	G only	No
4	G only	G and R	G and R	Yes

Based on these results, the researcher determined that estrogen had no effect when not bound to a cytosolic, estrogen-specific receptor.

Persuasive Reasoning

These passages typically present a scientific phenomenon along with a hypothesis that explains the phenomenon, and may include counter-arguments as well. Questions associated with these passages ask you to evaluate the hypothesis or arguments. Persuasive Reasoning passages in the science sections of the MCAT tend to be less common than Information Presentation or Experiment-based passages. Here is an example of a Persuasive Reasoning passage:

Two theoretical chemists attempted to explain the observed trends of acidity by applying two interpretations of molecular orbital theory. Consider the pK_a values of some common acids listed along with the conjugate base:

acid	pK_a	conjugate base
H_2SO_4	< 0	HSO_4^-
H_2CrO_4	5.0	$HCrO_4^-$
H_2PO_4	2.1	$H_2PO_4^-$
HF	3.9	F^-
HOCl	7.8	ClO^-
HCN	9.5	CN^-
HIO_3	1.2	IO_3^-

Recall that acids with a $pK_a < 0$ are called strong acids, and those with a $pK_a > 0$ are called weak acids. The arguments of the chemists are given below.

Chemist #1:

"The acidity of a compound is proportional to the polarization of the H—X bond, where X is some nonmetal element. Complex acids, such as H_2SO_4, $HClO_4$, and HNO_3 are strong acids because the H—O bonding electrons are strongly drawn towards the oxygen. It is generally true that a covalent bond weakens as its polarization increases. Therefore, one can conclude that the strength of an acid is proportional to the number of electronegative atoms in that acid."

Chemist #2:

"The acidity of a compound is proportional to the number of stable resonance structures of that acid's conjugate base. H_2SO_4, $HClO_4$, and HNO_3 are all strong acids because their respective conjugate bases exhibit a high degree of resonance stabilization."

MAPPING A PASSAGE

"Mapping a passage" refers to the combination of on-screen highlighting and scratch paper notes that you take while working through a passage. Typically, good things to highlight include the overall topic of a paragraph, unfamiliar terms, unusual terms, italicized terms, numerical values, hypothesis, and results. Scratch paper notes can be used to summarize the paragraphs and to jot down important facts and connections that are made when reading the passage. More details on passage mapping will be presented in Section 2.5.

2.3   GENERAL SCIENCE QUESTION TYPES

Questions in the science sections are generally one of three main types: Memory, Explicit, or Implicit.

Memory Questions

These questions can be answered directly from prior knowledge, with no need to reference the passage or question text. Memory questions represent approximately 25 percent of the science questions on the MCAT. Usually, Memory questions are found as FSQs, but they can also be tucked into a passage. Here's an example of a Memory question:

> Which of the following acetylating conditions will convert diethylamine into an amide at the fastest rate?
>
> A)   Acetic acid/HCl
> B)   Acetic anhydride
> C)   Acetyl chloride
> D)   Ethyl acetate

Explicit Questions

Explicit questions can be answered primarily with information from the passage, along with prior knowledge. They may require data retrieval, graph analysis, or making a simple connection. Explicit questions make up approximately 35–40 percent of the science questions on the MCAT; here's an example (taken from the sample Information/Situation Presentation passage):

> The sensor device D shown in Figure 1 performs its function by acting as:
>
> A)   an ohmmeter.
> B)   a voltmeter.
> C)   a potentiometer.
> D)   an ammeter.

Implicit Questions

These questions require you to take information from the passage, combine it with your prior knowledge, apply it to a new situation, and come to some logical conclusion. They typically require more complex connections than do Explicit questions, and may also require data retrieval, graph analysis, etc. Implicit questions usually require a solid understanding of the passage information. They make up approximately 35–40 percent of the science questions on the MCAT; here's an example (taken from the sample Experiment/Research Presentation passage):

> If Experiment 2 were repeated, but this time exposing the cells first to Pesticide A and then to Pesticide B before exposing them to the green fluorescent-labeled estrogen and the red fluorescent probe, which of the following statements will most likely be true?
>
> A) Pesticide A and Pesticide B bind to the same site on the estrogen receptor.
> B) Estrogen effects would be observed.
> C) Only green fluorescence would be observed.
> D) Both green and red fluorescence would be observed.

The Rod of Asclepius

You may notice this Rod of Asclepius icon as you read through the book. In Greek mythology, the Rod of Asclepius is associated with healing and medicine; the symbol continues to be used today to represent medicine and healthcare. You won't see this on the actual MCAT, but we've used it here to call attention to medically related examples and questions.

2.4   ORGANIC CHEMISTRY ON THE MCAT

The science sections of the MCAT have 10 passages and 15 freestanding questions (FSQs). Organic chemistry is the least prevalent subject tested on the MCAT, and will make up roughly 15% of the Chemical and Physical Foundations of Biological Systems section and only about 5% of the questions on the Biological and Biochemical Foundations of Living Systems section. In the Chemical and Physical Foundations section of the test, the questions will be distributed between two to four freestanding questions and either one longer passage (with five or six questions) or two very short passages (usually with four questions each). In the Biological and Biochemical Foundations section, the three or four O-Chem questions are likely to be either FSQs, or mixed in with either a biology or biochemistry passage. The O-Chem topics covered span roughly two college semesters' worth of material but focus most on carbonyl chemistry and laboratory techniques. For now, let's talk about what you can expect from O-Chem passages more generally, and we'll get to specific content in the coming chapters.

2.5 TACKLING AN ORGANIC CHEMISTRY PASSAGE

In general, some sort of biologically important compound or reaction provides the context for O-Chem passages. The text of the passage might contain biologically related concepts or facts, but a sure sign that you're reading an O-Chem passage and not a Biology passage will be chemical structures, usually lots of them.

Your approach to reading and mapping an O-Chem passage should be a bit different than your approach for all other subjects. The reason? There is hardly ever information within the text of an O-Chem passage that will be useful or needed to answer passage-based questions. The most important information in these passages will be in the form of chemical structures from synthetic or mechanistic schemes, or experimental data from a table, graph, or figure. Often, complicated syntheses and mechanisms can be intimidating because of all the detail presented, and they can slow you down considerably if you pay too much attention to this information during your first run through the passage. Be sure to read the titles of figures or schemes to get a sense of the big picture being presented, then jump into answering the questions quickly.

Passage Types as They Apply to Organic Chemistry

The main science passage types mentioned previously, when considered in the context of O-Chem, look something like this:

Information and/or Situation Presentation

These are the most common types of O-Chem passages, and generally present:

- A multistep synthetic scheme, a novel reaction, or atypical outcomes of reactions you might already be familiar with. Questions associated with these passages might ask you to analyze or classify the steps of the process described, or use common laboratory techniques to analyze intermediate compounds in the synthesis. You might need to justify the exceptions to the rules as described.

- A class of biologically important molecules. Questions associated with these passages could ask you to analyze the molecules with a common laboratory technique, or simply ask about their structure or their relationship to each other. You might also need to predict the reactivity of the molecules if treated with a given reagent.

- A biochemical process or mechanism. Questions here often test your understanding of the stability of intermediates and ask you to explain why the reaction occurs in the manner described. Given a new reactant, you might need to use the mechanistic steps to predict the product of a reaction.

Experiment/Research Presentation

This type of passage presents the details of an experiment or a mechanistic study, and often includes spectroscopy data (IR or NMR) in the form of lists or tables. Questions ask you to interpret data and identify the likely pathway of reaction. You might also need to identify compounds, or simply choose the appropriate technique to achieve the desired purification or product identification.

Persuasive Reasoning

This is the least common type of O-Chem passage, but can appear as a comparison of two mechanisms that attempt to explain the outcome of a reaction. Questions ask you to evaluate the arguments presented and will likely relate to the stability of intermediates.

2.5

Reading an O-Chem Passage

You should never really *read* much of the text of an O-Chem passage, but rather, just skim through the text. Remember that most of the important information you'll use from an O-Chem passage will be in the form of the structures and data presented. O-Chem passage-based questions are often essentially freestanding questions. They require only reference to a structure given in the passage in order to answer. However, as you're skimming the passage, you won't know which structures, reaction steps, or data will be the useful bits, AND you won't be able to mark or highlight structures in any way using your onscreen tools. That means that when skimming, you should get a general sense of the importance of each figure or table by reading titles and headings, but not get bogged down in the details of the figures in any way. You want to know where to go to examine the details when a question refers you to a particular synthetic step or structure along the pathway, something the MCAT is amazingly kind enough to do in most cases.

While you're reading, be on the lookout for new *italicized* terms in the text to highlight, or unexpected outcomes of experiments and exceptions to rules. The MCAT will ask you to apply the science fundamentals you've studied to novel situations, so look for and highlight anything that might be out of the ordinary.

Mapping an O-Chem Passage

It will often be the case that the text of a passage will reproduce information presented in a more visually useful manner, such as a flowchart, reaction scheme, or mechanism. Try to focus on the structures, and resist the urge to make a lot of yellow marks in the text.

Since you cannot highlight any structures in the passage (this is unfortunate, since structures are the place you'll get most of your necessary information), remember to use your scratch paper to make note of anything related to a reaction scheme or mechanism, especially if it's taken you some time to come to your conclusion. Keep your scratch paper organized so it will be a useful tool if you need to refer to it while checking back over your answers toward the end of the section. Label each new passage with a number on your paper and the range of questions attached to that passage, and give it an identifying title that summarizes the main point of the passage.

If you reach an important conclusion while answering questions, be sure to make note of it on your scratch paper too. Other questions may require this information in order to proceed, and a brief note beats wasted time reconfirming your conclusion while trying to answer a subsequent question. Your O-Chem passage map will begin to develop as you answer your questions, but before jumping into answering them, you will likely have very little to jot down.

The passage below is an example of an Information Presentation passage (of the second type described previously). Note the minimal highlighting. The highlighted text was seemingly important upon a first pass to identify what the passage was about and to predict the types of questions with which it might be associated. You'll find upon review of the questions, however, that nothing but structures was necessary to answer any of the passage-based questions.

The small milkweed bug, *Lygaeus kalmii*, produces and emits a number of C_5-C_8 alkenals. Some of these small, fragrant, organic molecules are used to attract conspecific males or females for mating; thus, they act as sex pheromones. Others of the molecules are strongly malodorous and are used for defense.

Collaborating scientists in Brazil, the Netherlands, and Maryland have recently developed a method of noninvasive sampling and identification of these small organic molecules from live insects. This method involves the use of gas chromatography and mass spectrometry for the separation and identification of the components of the mixture of molecules involved in the sex- and defense-pheromone response in *L. kalmii*. Several of the molecules identified in this manner are shown in Figure 1.

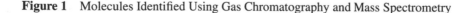

(*E*)-2-Hexenal

(*E*,*E*)-2,4-Octadienal

4-Oxo-(*E*)-2-Octenal

Figure 1 Molecules Identified Using Gas Chromatography and Mass Spectrometry

2.5

In addition to its mass spectrum, Molecule A, shown below, was also identified by its ^{1}H NMR spectrum:

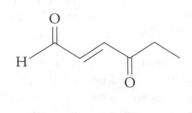

Molecule A

Remember not to get bogged down in spectroscopic data before a question specifically asks you to analyze it. Here is an example of a passage map for the passage above. This is what you might jot down on your scratch paper:

P1 – alkenals
P2 – separation and identification of alkenals
P3 – NMR data

The passage below is another example of an Information Presentation passage (of the third type described previously). While the passage has much more text to wade through, only one small piece of it proves to be important in an Explicit question (addressed in detail later). Highlighted items are related to the main point of each paragraph, include new definitions, or provide examples of phenomena. The figures presented are more complex than those in the first passage, and the questions related to them are likely to be more involved as well.

Dyes are ionizable, aromatic compounds that absorb visible light due to the presence of a highly conjugated system of p orbitals. The observed color is one that is complementary to the wavelength of light absorbed by the molecule (complementary color pairs are red/green, orange/blue, and yellow/violet). Dyes bind to the materials to be colored, such as fabrics or paper, through inter- and intramolecular interactions, including hydrogen bonds, ionic interactions, covalent bonds, and coordinate covalent bonds. The stronger the interaction between dye molecule and fiber, the more permanent the color will be. When a dye covalently bonds to a fiber, it becomes a part of the fabric itself and cannot be washed away.

Two of the most common dye types are mordant dyes and direct dyes. A mordant is a polyvalent metal ion (usually Al^{3+} or Fe^{3+}) that forms a coordination complex with certain dyes. Mordants chelate to the fabric as well as the dye molecule, thereby improving their colorfastness. Mordant dyes are primarily used on protein-based fibers such as wool, silk, angora, and cashmere since the mordant can bind to the constituent amino acids of these fibers. Direct dyes are typically charged molecules, and interact with the material to be dyed through ionic forces or hydrogen bonding. As such they tend to bleed more than mordant dyes. Direct dyes are more commonly used on cellulose fibers such as cotton, linen, or hemp.

Azo dyes, a subclass of direct dyes, may be used in a dyeing technique in which an insoluble azo compound is produced directly onto or within a fiber. This is achieved by treating the fiber first with a diazonium component, followed by a coupling component. With suitable adjustment of dye bath conditions the two components react to produce the required insoluble azo dye. The coupling reagent used in the final step is typically a molecule containing either a phenolic hydroxyl group or an arylamine. The synthesis of methyl orange, an azo dye, is shown in Figure 1.

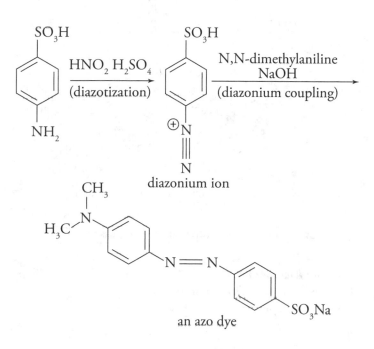

Figure 1 Synthesis of methyl orange

Figure 2 below represents the mechanism of the diazonium coupling reaction in the synthesis of methyl orange.

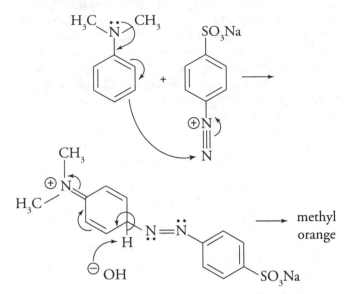

Figure 2 Mechanism of diazonium coupling

This is what you might jot down on your scratch paper for the passage above:

P1 – what dyes are and how they work
P2 – Definitions: mordant dye vs. direct dyes, fiber types dyed
P3 – Structure requirements for diazocoupling

2.6 TACKLING THE QUESTIONS

The Organic Chemistry passage-based questions are some of the most straightforward ones on the entire exam and, as a result, some of the quickest ones to answer. It may be a wise strategy to consider doing the O-Chem passages before the Biology, Physics, or General Chemistry ones to help bank up some extra time to spend on the wordier, more involved Biology passages.

However, you should also consider starting with whichever subject you feel the most comfortable with, saving your more difficult subject for last. Whatever subject you choose, do all of the passages in one subject first before switching. In addition, do the passages within a subject in the order with which you feel most comfortable, leaving the topic you struggle with most, or the passage that appears to be the most difficult, for last. Within the passages themselves, tackle the easier questions first, leaving the most time consuming ones for last. See Chapter 1, "MCAT Basics" for more information on effeciently moving around in the test.

O-Chem Memory Questions

These questions can be answered directly from prior knowledge. You can often recognize this question type by the length of the answer choices; one- or two-word answer choices are a good indication that you have the answer to these questions in your head already. Freestanding questions are commonly Memory questions since there is no passage to refer to. In addition, O-Chem passages often have "hidden" FSQs associated with them. This is another good reason to get to the questions quickly, rather than getting stuck reading details within the passage text.

Here is a true freestanding question that is also a Memory question:

> Which of the following acetylating conditions will convert diethylamine into an amide at the fastest rate?
>
> A) Acetic acid/HCl
> B) Acetic anhydride
> C) Acetyl chloride
> D) Ethyl acetate

Your first step to attacking this question should be to consider what type of reaction is described. The conversion of an amine to an amide is a nucleophilic addition-elimination, where the amine acts as the nucleophile. Therefore, you're looking for the answer choice with the best electrophile, thereby increasing the reaction rate. Knowing the relative reactivities of carboxylic acids derivatives (amide < ester < anhydride < acid halide) allows you to eliminate choices B and D. In order to choose between the remaining answers that include a carboxylic acid and an acid derivative, rely on your fundamentals. Ask yourself: How would an amine be expected to behave under each set of conditions? When you consider that amines are not only nucleophilic but also basic, you can deduce that they will be protonated by both the HCl and the acetic acid to yield a non-nucleophilic conjugate acid under the conditions of answer choice A. The nucleophilic addition reaction is therefore faster with the acid chloride derivative, making answer choice C correct.

O-Chem Explicit Questions

These questions have answers that are explicitly stated in the passage. To answer them correctly, for example, may just require finding a definition, reading a graph, or making a simple connection. Explicit questions are much more common in passages of the test that rely more on reading comprehension. Since chemical structures are the most common source of referenced information in an O-Chem passage, Explicit questions in this section might ask you to identify the number of chiral centers in a given molecule, or to identify whether a particular functional group is present or not.

Here's an example of an Explicit question from the azo dye passage:

> Mordant dyes are used in biological assays in addition to the textile industry. Which of the following biologically important molecules is most likely to be labeled by a mordant dye?
>
> A) Glycogen
> B) Chromatin
> C) Cholesterol
> D) Starch

You should recognize the term "mordant" as a new term you highlighted while reading the passage, so go back to the text to retrieve the important information. The passage states that mordants generally bind to protein-based fibers. Without this information, you might be able to eliminate choices A and D (glycogen and starch) since they are both carbohydrates, and as such, are not likely to be the answer. With the passage information at your disposal, however, this becomes a bit of a Memory question, and you need only determine which of your answer choices contain proteins. Cholesterol, a lipid, can be eliminated in addition to the two carbohydrates, leaving choice B as the correct answer (note that chromatin contains both proteins and DNA).

O-Chem Implicit Questions

These questions require you to apply knowledge to a new situation or make a more complex connection; the answer is typically implied by the information in the passage. Answer choices are generally longer, and may come in two parts, where the second half provides an explanation for the first. As mentioned before, the relevant information in the passage is often a molecular structure, but the analysis required to answer the question is more involved than for Explicit questions that rely on structures. Implicit style questions are the most common types of O-Chem questions.

Here's an example of an Implicit question from the azo dye passage:

> The diazonium coupling reaction in Figure 2 is faster than most electrophilic substitutions of benzene. Which of the following statements best explains this fact?
>
> A) The diazonium ion is an electron withdrawing substituent, making its benzene ring a better electrophile than benzene.
> B) The diazonium ion is a good nucleophile.
> C) The dimethylamino group is an electron donating substituent, making its benzene ring a better electrophile than benzene.
> D) The dimethylamino group is an electron donating substituent, making its benzene ring a better nucleophile than benzene.

Since these answer choices are relatively long (and most have a second clause), try to use POE to eliminate choices based on obvious false statements in the first part of the answer. Remember, if any part of an answer choice is false, the entire statement can be eliminated. The first half of all the choices makes a statement about the inductive effects of substituents, or, in the case of answer choice B, the nucleophilicity of a compound. Refer to the structures in Figure 2. You should note that the diazonium ion is positively charged and therefore electron deficient. Since nucleophiles are by definition electron rich, choice B can be eliminated. The first halves of the remaining answer choices are all valid statements, since a positively charged substituent will pull electron density toward it, while an amine with a lone pair of electrons on the nitrogen will push electron density toward the ring. This question requires a more critical approach to distinguish between answer choices.

You should identify this as an Implicit question since it asks you to compare a new reagent to one you might already be familiar with. Consider, then, what you already know about benzene. Since benzene has six π electrons and is electron rich, it should behave as a nucleophile. This fundamental piece of information about the reactivity of benzene allows you to eliminate choices A and C. It does not matter whether the indicated substituents in Figure 2 make benzene a better or worse electrophile, since in the context of this reaction benzene behaves as a nucleophile. The remaining answer (choice D) is not only internally consistent but also answers the question.

Content Categories

O-Chem questions can be further classified from a content perspective into four main categories. Instead of trying to memorize a lot of detailed information, try to generalize as much as possible, and focus on the fundamentals of structure and stability when approaching questions. Remember that the MCAT is more likely to ask you to apply fundamental concepts to novel situations rather than ask you to recall an exception to a rule and regurgitate trivia. Just about every O-Chem question can be put into one of the following five categories:

Structure

Questions are generally about functional groups, stereochemistry, isomers, electron density (nucleophiles vs. electrophiles), and nomenclature.

Stability

This generally refers to stability of products or reaction intermediates. These questions often ask about inductive effects, resonance, steric strain, torsional strain, ring strain, etc.

Laboratory practices

These questions may ask you to identify an appropriate separation technique (extraction, chromatography, distillation, etc.) for a given mixture of compounds, or ask you to interpret/predict the results of a separation procedure. You might also be asked to choose an appropriate spectroscopic technique (IR, NMR, mass spec, UV-vis, etc.) to identify a compound, or interpret spectroscopic data.

Predict the product

Given a starting material and reaction conditions, choose the major product of the reaction. This will only be a one step synthesis; no multi-step processes will be presented. These questions will generally be associated with a passage in which a reaction type is explained in detail rather than be a freestanding question.

Finally, let's take a look at some sound advice about how to manage your time effectively while answering individual questions, as well as good strategies or rules of thumb you can apply to attack some of the most common formats of questions you'll see on the MCAT.

ORGANIC CHEMISTRY QUESTION STRATEGIES

1. Remember that Process of Elimination is paramount! The strikeout tool allows you to eliminate answer choices; this will improve your chances of guessing the correct answer if you are unable to narrow it down to one choice.

2. Answer the straightforward questions first. Leave questions that require analysis of experiments and graphs for later.

3. Make sure that the answer you choose actually answers the question, and isn't just a true statement.

4. I-II-III questions: Always work between the I-II-III statements and the answer choices. Unfortunately, it is not possible to strike out the Roman numerals, but this is a great use for scratch paper notes. Once a statement is determined to be true (or false), strike out answer choices that do not contain (or do contain) that statement as appropriate.

5. Ranking questions: Look for an extreme in whatever is being ranked, then look at the answer choices. Use the strikeout feature to eliminate choices as you go. In some cases, you may immediately get the answer as only one choice lists the appropriate option as "least" or "greatest." Usually you will, at minimum, be able to strikeout two answer choices. Then just examine the remaining possibilities to determine which of the items at the other end of the ranking can be correct.

6. 2 x 2 style questions: These questions require you to know two pieces of information to get the correct answer, and are easily identified by their answer choices, which commonly take the form A because X, B because X, A because Y, B because Y. Tackle one piece of information at a time, which should allow you to quickly eliminate two answer choices.

7. LEAST/EXCEPT/NOT questions: Don't get tricked by these questions that ask you to pick the answer that doesn't fit (the incorrect or false statement). It's often good to use your scratch paper and write a T or F next to answer choices A–D. The one that stands out as different is the correct answer!

8. If you read a question and do not know how to answer it, look to the passage for help. It is likely that the passage contains information pertinent to answering the question, either within the text or in the form of experimental data.

9. Math: Any questions that involve calculations should be left for last (there aren't many in O-Chem, but they happen). You should always round numbers and estimate while working out calculations on your scratch paper.

10. Don't ever leave a question blank since there is no penalty for guessing.

Chapter 3
Organic Chemistry Fundamentals

3.1 BACKGROUND AND INTRODUCTION

This section covers the fundamentals of nomenclature in organic chemistry. Although this section will require memorization as your primary study technique, it is in your best interest to be comfortable reading, hearing, and using this terminology. Although most of the terminology that appears on the MCAT is IUPAC, some common nomenclature is also used.

Basic Nomenclature

Carbon Chain Prefixes and Alkane Names			
Number of carbon atoms in a row	Prefix	Alkane	Name
1	meth-	CH_4	methane
2	eth-	CH_3CH_3	ethane
3	prop-	$CH_3CH_2CH_3$	propane
4	but-	$CH_3CH_2CH_2CH_3$	butane
5	pent-	$CH_3(CH_2)_3CH_3$	pentane
6	hex-	$CH_3(CH_2)_4CH_3$	hexane
7	hept-	$CH_3(CH_2)_5CH_3$	heptane
8	oct-	$CH_3(CH_2)_6CH_3$	octane
9	non-	$CH_3(CH_2)_7CH_3$	nonane
10	dec-	$CH_3(CH_2)_8CH_3$	decane

In the case of an all-carbon containing ring, these are preceded by the prefix **cyclo-**. Hence, a six-membered ring containing all $-CH_2-$ units is called *cyclohexane*.

Nomenclature For Substituents	
Substituent	Name
$-CH_3$	methyl
$-CH_2CH_3$	ethyl
$-CH_2CH_2CH_3$	propyl
$H_3C-\overset{\displaystyle H}{\underset{\displaystyle |}{C}}-CH_3$	isopropyl
$-CH_2CH_2CH_2CH_3$	butyl (or *n*-butyl)
$CH_3\underset{\displaystyle |}{C}HCH_2CH_3$	*sec*-butyl
$\overset{\displaystyle CH_3}{\underset{\displaystyle CH_3}{-\overset{\displaystyle |}{\underset{\displaystyle |}{C}}-CH_3}}$	*tert*-butyl (or *t*-butyl)

Common Functional Groups

R = alkyl group   X = halogen (F, Cl, Br, I)

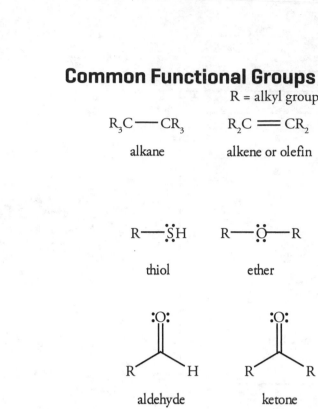

R_3C—CR_3

alkane

R_2C=CR_2

alkene or olefin

RC≡CR

alkyne

R—X

alkyl halide

R—$\ddot{O}H$

alcohol

R—$\ddot{S}H$

thiol

R—$\ddot{O}$—R

ether

epoxide or oxirane

phenol

aldehyde

ketone

hemiacetal

acetal

cyanohydrin

amine

imine

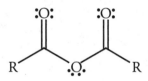
enamine

carboxylic acid

acid halide

acid anhydride

ester

lactone

amide

lactam

3.2 ABBREVIATED LINE STRUCTURES

The prevalence of carbon-hydrogen (C—H) bonds in organic chemistry has led chemists to use an abbreviated drawing system, merely for convenience. Just imagine having to draw every C—H bond for a large molecule like a steroid or polymer! Abbreviated line structures use only a few simple rules:

1. Carbons are represented simply as vertices.
2. C—H bonds are not drawn.
3. Hydrogens bonded to any atom *other* than carbon must be shown.

To illustrate rules 1 and 2, pentane can be represented using the full Lewis structure,

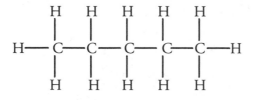

or using the abbreviated line structure.

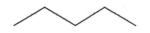

Although C—H bonds are not drawn, the number of hydrogens required to complete carbon's valency are assumed. To clarify this, let's look more closely at the abbreviated line structure of pentane:

These three carbon atoms are each bonded to two other carbon atoms. In order to complete carbon's valency, we assume there are two hydrogens bonded to each of these carbons.

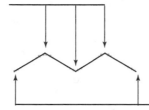

These two carbon atoms are each bonded to one other carbon atom. In order to complete carbon's valency, we assume there are three hydrogens bonded to each of these carbons.

This must be correct, because if we draw out all of the hydrogens in pentane, we get the full Lewis structure shown above.

To illustrate rule 3, consider dimethyl amine:

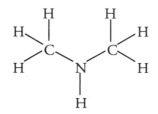

full Lewis structure

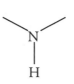

abbreviated line
structure

Remember that hydrogens bonded to carbon can be assumed (the methyl groups in dimethyl amine, for example), but hydrogens bonded to any other atom must be shown. Lone pairs of electrons are often omitted.

Example 3-1: Translate each of the following Lewis structures into an abbreviated line structure:

(a)

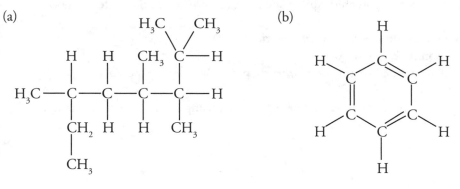

(b)

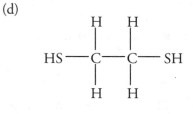

(c)

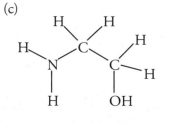

(d)

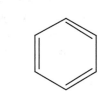

Solution:

(a)

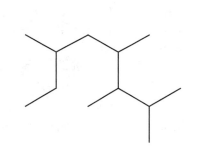

(b)

(c)

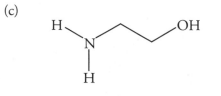

(d)

Example 3-2: Translate each of the following abbreviated line structures into a Lewis structure:

(a)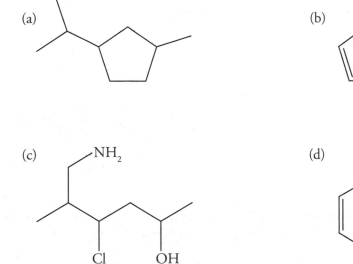

(b)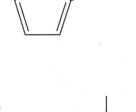

(c)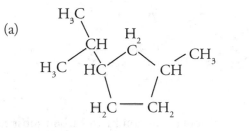

(d)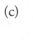

Solution:

(a)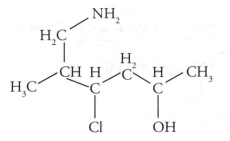

(b)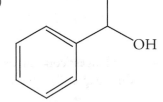

(c)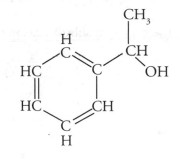

(d)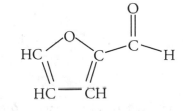

3.3 NOMENCLATURE OF ALKANES

Alkanes are named by a set of simple rules. One particular alkane (shown below) will be used to illustrate this process:

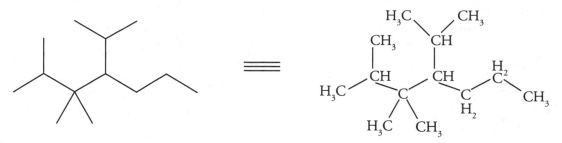

1. Identify the longest continuous carbon chain. The names of these chains are given in the first table in this chapter ("Carbon Chain Prefixes and Alkane Names").

    The longest chain in the compound above is a 7-carbon chain, which is called *heptane*. (This chain is shown below, outlined by dashed lines.)

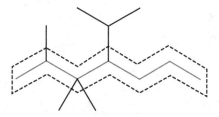

2. Identify any substituents on this chain. The names of some common hydrocarbon substituents are given in the second table in this chapter ("Nomenclature for Substituents").

    There are four substituents in this example: three methyl groups and one isopropyl group.

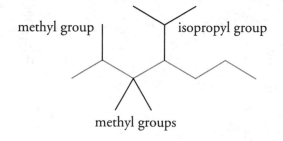

3. Number the carbons of the main chain such that the substituents are on the carbons with lower numbers.

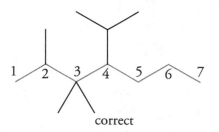

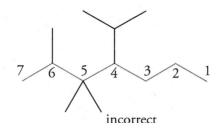

Now each substituent can be associated with the carbon atom to which it's attached:

2 – methyl
3 – methyl
3 – methyl
4 – isopropyl

4. Identical substituents are grouped together; the prefixes **di-**, **tri-**, **tetra-**, and **penta-** are used to denote how many there are, and their carbon numbers are separated by a comma.

In this case we have

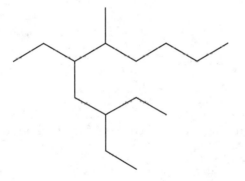

2 – methyl
3 – methyl ⟶ 2,3,3-trimethyl
3 – methyl

5. Alphabetize the substituents, ignoring the prefixes di-, tri-, etc. and *n-*, *sec-*, *tert-*, and separate numbers from words by a hyphen and numbers from numbers by a comma. Note that "iso" is not a prefix but is part of the name of the substituent, so it is NOT ignored when alphabetizing.

The complete name for our molecule is therefore **4-isopropyl-2,3,3-trimethylheptane.**

Let's do another example and find the name of this molecule:

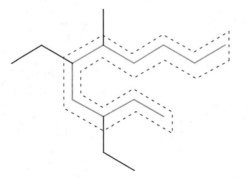

1. The longest continuous carbon chain is a 10-carbon chain, called **decane**.

2. There are three substituents on this chain: two ethyl groups and a methyl group.

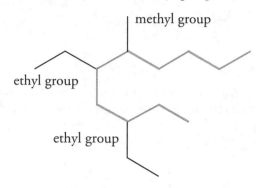

3. The correct numbering of the carbons in the main chain is as follows:

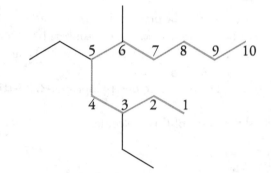

4. The substituents are now identified as:
    3,5-diethyl
    6-methyl

5. The complete name of the molecule is therefore **3,5-diethyl-6-methyldecane**.

Example 3-3: Name each of the following alkanes:

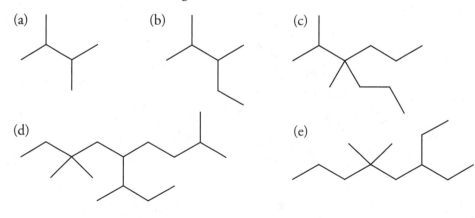

Solution:

(a) 2,3-dimethylbutane
(b) 2,3-dimethylpentane
(c) 4-isopropyl-4-methylheptane
(d) 5-*sec*-butyl-2,7,7-trimethylnonane
(e) 3-ethyl-5,5-dimethyloctane

3.4 NOMENCLATURE OF HALOALKANES

Alkanes with halogen (F, Cl, Br, I) substituents follow the same set of rules as simple alkanes. Halogens are named using these prefixes:

Halogen	Prefix
fluorine	fluoro-
chlorine	chloro-
bromine	bromo-
iodine	iodo-

By applying the same rules as for naming simple alkanes, verify the following names:

Structure   Name

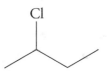 2-chlorobutane

2-chloro-1-fluoro-4-methylpentane

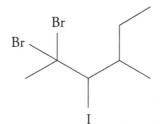 2,2-dibromo-3-iodo-4-methylhexane

3.4

Example 3-4: Name each of the following haloalkanes:

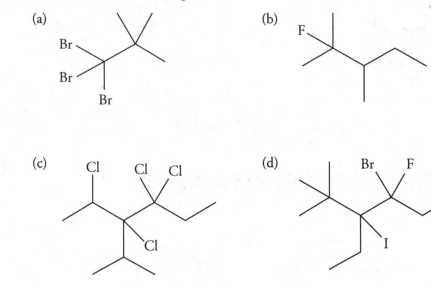

Solution:

(a) 1,1,1-tribromo-2,2-dimethylpropane
(b) 2-fluoro-2,3-dimethylpentane
(c) 2,3,4,4-tetrachloro-3-isopropylhexane
(d) 4-bromo-3-ethyl-4-fluoro-3-iodo-2,2-dimethylhexane

Example 3-5: For each name, draw the structure:

(a) 3-chloro-2,2-dimethylbutane
(b) 3-bromo-4-chloro-5,5-diethylnonane
(c) 2,3-dibromo-1,1-diiodopropane
(d) 3,4-difluoro-2,2,3-trimethylpentane

Solution:

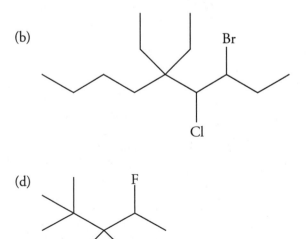

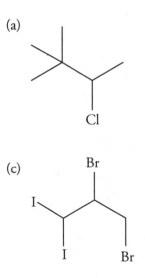

3.5   NOMENCLATURE OF ALCOHOLS

Alcohols also follow many of the same nomenclature rules as alkanes. Hydroxyl groups (–OH), however, are typically denoted by a suffix to the main alkyl chain. The table of straight-chain alcohols given below shows that to denote a hydroxyl group, the suffix **–ol** replaces the last **–e** in the name of the alkane.

Alkanes		Alcohols	
Structure	Name	Structure	Name
CH_4	methane	CH_3OH	methanol
CH_3CH_3	ethane	CH_3CH_2OH	ethanol
$CH_3CH_2CH_3$	propane	$CH_3CH_2CH_2OH$	propanol
$CH_3CH_2CH_2CH_3$	butane	$CH_3CH_2CH_2CH_2OH$	butanol

When the position of the hydroxyl group needs to be specified, the number is placed after the name of the longest carbon chain and before the –ol suffix, separated by hyphens. For example:

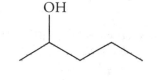

butan-2-ol
(or 2-butanol)
or *sec*-butanol

pentan-2-ol
(or 2-pentanol)

Priorities are assigned (the way the main carbon chain is numbered) to give the lowest number to the hydroxyl group. For example:

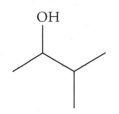

3-methylbutan-2-ol
not
2-methylbutan-3-ol

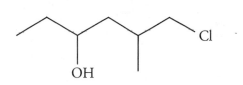

6-chloro-5-methylhexan-3-ol

Example 3-6: Name each of the following molecules:

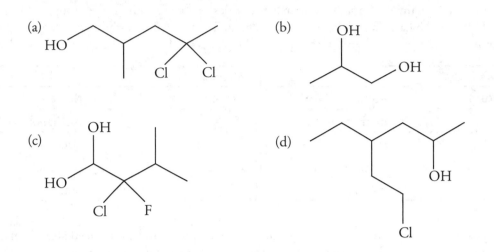

(a)
(b)
(c)
(d)

Solution:

(a) 4,4-dichloro-2-methylpentanol (the "-1-" is assumed if no number is given)
(b) propane-1,2-diol (or 1,2-propandiol)
(c) 2-chloro-2-fluoro-3-methylbutane-1,1-diol
(d) 6-chloro-4-ethylhexan-2-ol

Other organic functional groups have small nuances to their nomenclature, but this introduction to nomenclature should allow you to interpret chemical names on the MCAT.

Chapter 4
Structure and Stability

4.1 THE ORGANIC CHEMIST'S TOOLBOX

In the following chapters, we will frequently discuss several fundamental principles necessary to understand the reactivity of organic molecules. These "tools" are collected here.

Structural Formulas

By definition, an organic molecule is said to be **saturated** if it contains no π bonds and no rings; it is **unsaturated** if it has at least one π bond or a ring. A saturated compound with *n* carbon atoms has exactly 2*n* + 2 hydrogen atoms, while an unsaturated compound with *n* carbon atoms has fewer than 2*n* + 2 hydrogens.

The formula below is used to determine the **degree of unsaturation** (*d*) of simple organic molecules:

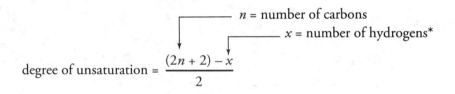

$$\text{degree of unsaturation} = \frac{(2n + 2) - x}{2}$$

n = number of carbons
x = number of hydrogens*

* *x* represents the number of hydrogens and any monovalent
atoms (such as the halogens: F, Cl, Br, or I).
Since the number of oxygens has no effect, it is ignored.
For nitrogen-containing compounds, replace each N by
1 C and 1 H when using this formula.

One degree of unsaturation indicates the presence of one π bond or one ring; two degrees of unsaturation means there are two π bonds (two separate double bonds or one triple bond), or one π bond and one ring, or two rings, and so on. The presence of heteroatoms can also affect the degree of unsaturation in a molecule. This is best illustrated through a series of related molecules that all have one degree of unsaturation.

Butene (C_4H_8) has one degree of unsaturation, since $d = [(2 \times 4 + 2) - 8]/2 = 1$, in the form of a double bond:

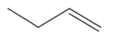

4-Chlorobutene (C_4H_7Cl) also has one degree of unsaturation, but the number of hydrogens is different. Each halogen atom (fluorine, chlorine, bromine, iodine) or other monovalent atom "replaces" one hydrogen atom, so $d = [(2 \times 4 + 2) - (7 + 1)]/2 = 1$:

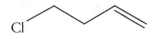

Methoxyethene (C_3H_6O) also has one degree of unsaturation. Since a divalent atom can take the place of a methylene group, it doesn't affect the degree of unsaturation, and can be ignored. The calculation for this formula, then, should look like this: $[(2 \times 3 + 2) - 6]/2 = 1$

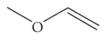

Methyl vinyl amine (C_3H_7N) has one degree of unsaturation as well. Each nitrogen (or other trivalent atom) "replaces" one carbon and one hydrogen atom. Therefore, adjust the formula to be C_4H_8, then do the calculation. The new formula thus gives $d = [(2 \times 4 + 2) - 8]/2 = 1$:

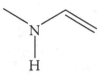

Example 4-1: Determine the degree of unsaturation of each of these molecules. Which, if any, are saturated?

(a) C_6H_8
(b) C_4H_6O
(c) $C_{20}H_{30}O$
(d) C_3H_8O
(e) C_3H_5Br

Solution:

(a) $d = [(2 \times 6 + 2) - 8]/2 = 3$.
(b) Just ignore the O, and find that $d = [(2 \times 4 + 2) - 6]/2 = 2$.
(c) Ignoring the O, we get $d = [(2 \times 20 + 2) - 30]/2 = 6$.
(d) Ignore the O, and find that $d = [(2 \times 3 + 2) - 8]/2 = 0$. *This molecule is saturated.*
(e) Since Br is a halogen, we treat it like a hydrogen, so $d = [(2 \times 3 + 2) - (5 + 1)]/2 = 1$.

Hybridization

Although hybridization theory is covered in more detail in the *MCAT General Chemistry Review*, it's useful here to briefly outline how to determine an atom's hybridization.

Every pair of electrons must be housed in an electronic orbital (either an *s, p, d,* or *f*). For example, the carbon atom in methane, CH_4, has *four* pairs of electrons surrounding it (four single covalent bonds and no lone pairs) so it must provide *four* orbitals to house these electrons. Orbitals always get "used" in the following order:

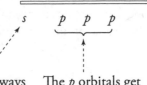

The single *s* orbital always gets used first.

The *p* orbitals get used up next. There are three *p* orbitals that may be used.

So, since the carbon atom in methane must provide *four* orbitals, we just count: 1…2…3…4:

Therefore, the hybridization of the carbon atom in methane is $s + p + p + p$, which is written as sp^3. The sum of the exponents in the hybridization nomenclature tells us how many orbitals of this type are used. So, in methane, there are $1 + 3 = 4$ hybrid orbitals. The following table gives the hybridization of the central atom for each of the orbital geometries:

Number of Electron Groups	Orbital Geometry	Hybridization of Central Atom
2	Linear	sp
3	Trigonal Planar	sp^2
4	Tetrahedral	sp^3

Reaction Intermediates

Some organic reactions proceed through carbocations (carbonium ions), while others make use of carbanions.

Carbocations, or **carbonium ions**, are positively charged species with a full positive charge on carbon. The reactivity of these species is determined by what type of carbon bears the positive charge. On the MCAT, carbocations will always be sp^2 hybridized with an empty *p* orbital.

Carbanions are negatively charged species with a full negative charge localized on carbon. The reactivity of these species is determined by what type of carbon bears the negative charge.

Stability Continuum				
Carbocations	3°	2°	1°	methyl
Carbanions	methyl	1°	2°	3°
	more stable	→		less stable
	less reactive	→		more reactive
	lower energy	→		higher energy

It's essential to understand the stabilities of reaction intermediates, because generally the reactivity of a molecule is inversely related to its stability. This means the molecules that are more stable are less reactive, while higher energy species will be more reactive. This theme will resurface over and over again in organic chemistry, and is a useful rule of thumb to keep in mind when you need to predict how a reaction might proceed.

Organic intermediates are stabilized in two major ways: **Inductive effects** stabilize charge through σ bonds, while **resonance effects** stabilize charge by delocalization through π bonds.

Inductive Effects

All substituent groups surrounding a reaction intermediate can be thought of as electron-withdrawing groups or electron-donating groups. **Electron-withdrawing** groups pull electrons toward themselves through σ bonds. **Electron-donating** groups donate (push) electron density away from themselves through σ bonds. Groups *more* electronegative than carbon tend to withdraw, while groups *less* electronegative than carbon tend to donate. On the MCAT, alkyl substituents are always electron-donating groups.

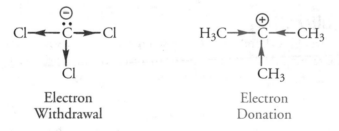

Electron-donating groups tend to stabilize electron-deficient intermediates (carbocations), while electron-withdrawing groups tend to stabilize electron-rich intermediates (carbanions). The stabilization of reaction intermediates by the sharing of electrons through σ bonds is called the **inductive effect**.

Example 4-2: Inductive effects frequently alter the reactivity of molecules. Justify the fact that trichloroacetic acid ($pK_a = 0.6$) is a better acid than acetic acid ($pK_a = 4.8$).

Solution: The chlorine atoms in trichloroacetic acid are electron withdrawing. This decreases the amount of electron density elsewhere in the molecule, especially in the O–H bond. With less electron density, the O–H bond is weaker, making it more acidic than the O–H bond in acetic acid.

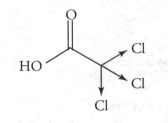

An alternative explanation would be to consider the stability of the conjugate bases of these acids.

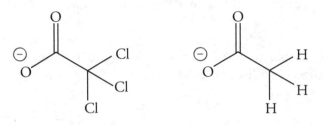

The chlorine atoms in the trichloroacetate anion distribute the negative charge better, making it more stable than the acetate anion. Therefore, because trichloroacetate anion is a weaker base (is more stable) than acetate anion, trichloroacetic acid is a stronger acid than acetic acid. Acidity will be reviewed in more detail a bit later in the Toolbox.

Resonance Stabilization

While induction works through σ bonds, resonance stabilization occurs in conjugated π systems. A **conjugated system** is one containing three or more atoms that each bear a p orbital. These orbitals are aligned so they are all parallel, creating the possibility of delocalized electrons.

Electrons that are confined to one orbital, either a bonding orbital between two atoms or a lone-pair orbital, are said to be **localized**. When electrons are allowed to interact with orbitals on adjacent atoms, they are no longer confined to their original "space," and so are termed **delocalized**. Consider the allyl cation:

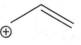

The electrons in the π bond can interact with the empty *p* orbital on the carbon bearing the positive charge. This is illustrated by the following resonance structures:

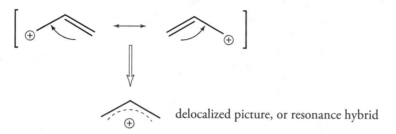

 delocalized picture, or resonance hybrid

The electron density is spread out—delocalized—over the entire 3-carbon framework in order to stabilize the carbocation. So, we might say of the allyl cation that both the electrons and the positive charge are delocalized.

As the allyl cation demonstrates, it often happens that a single Lewis structure for a molecule is not sufficient to most accurately represent the molecule's true structure. It is important to remember that resonance structures are just multiple representations of the actual structure. The molecule does not become one resonance structure or another; it exists as a combination of all resonance structures, although all may not contribute equally. All resonance structures must be drawn to give an accurate picture of the real nature of the molecule. In the case of the allyl cation, the two structures are equivalent and will have equivalent energy. They will also contribute equally to the delocalized picture of what the molecule really looks like. This average of all resonance contributors is called the **resonance hybrid**.

Benzene (C_6H_6) is another common molecule that exhibits resonance. Looking at a Lewis representation of benzene might lead one to believe that there are two distinct types of carbon-carbon bonds: single σ bonds (this structure of benzene has three such bonds) and double bonds (of which there are also three):

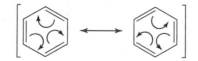

benzene

Thus one might expect two distinct carbon-carbon bond lengths: one for the single bonds, and one for the double bonds. Yet experimental data clearly demonstrate that all the C—C bond lengths are identical in benzene. All the carbons of benzene are sp^2 hybridized, so they each have an unhybridized *p* orbital. Two structures can be drawn for benzene, which differ only in the location of the π bonds. The true structure of benzene is best pictured as a resonance hybrid of these structures. Perhaps a better representation of benzene shows both resonance contributors, like this:

Notice that these resonance structures differ only in the arrangement of their π electrons, not in the locations of the atoms. All six unhybridized *p* orbitals are aligned parallel with one another. This alignment of adjacent unhybridized *p* orbitals allows for delocalization of π electrons over the entire ring. Whenever we have a delocalized π system (aligned *p* orbitals), resonance structures can be drawn.

Delocalization of electrons is also observed in thiophene:

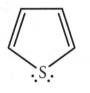

Here the sulfur atom has two pairs of non-bonding electrons. Notice that these electrons are one atom away from two π bonds. One pair of these electrons is actually in an unhybridized *p* orbital, such that it can be delocalized into the cyclic π system. Here are the representative resonance structures:

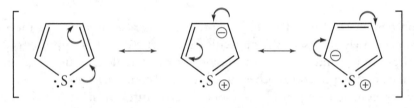

The other pair of electrons, however, is in a hybrid orbital and cannot delocalize into the π system. Here the delocalization of sulfur's electrons imparts aromatic stability to the molecule. The hybridization of the sulfur is therefore most correctly represented as *sp*².

Let's consider one more example:

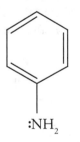

The nitrogen in aniline has an unshared electron pair that is one atom removed from a cyclic π system. Again these electrons can be delocalized by overlap of the lone pair-containing orbital with the *p* orbitals of the benzene ring. This can be demonstrated by the following resonance structures:

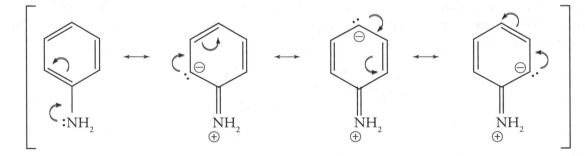

In this case, the delocalization of the nitrogen's electrons disrupts the aromaticity of the benzene ring and is therefore less favorable. Experimental determination of the nitrogen's bond angles reveals that they are actually intermediate between 120° and 109°, so the hybridization of the nitrogen can best be described not as sp^2 or sp^3, but as something intermediate between them. The important point, however, is that the electrons are at least somewhat delocalized into the π system. Therefore, the nitrogen's hybridization is not strictly sp^3.

Example 4-3: For the following molecules, indicate the hybridization and idealized bond angles for the indicated atoms.

(a)

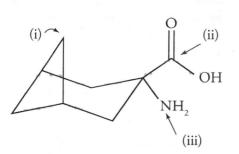

(b)

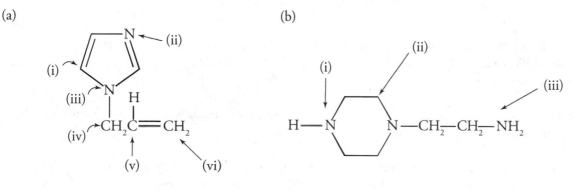

(c)

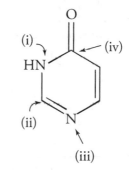

(d)

(e)

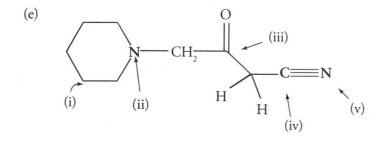

(f)

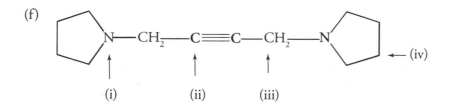

Solution: Remember to always draw the electrons on nitrogen if they are not drawn in the structure.

(a) i) sp^2, 120°   ii) sp^2, 120°   iii) sp^2, 120° (The lone pair is delocalized, so it's not counted.)
      iv) sp^3, 109°   v) sp^2, 120°   vi) sp^2, 120°

(b) i) sp^3, 109°   ii) sp^3, 109°   iii) sp^3, 109°

(c) i) sp^3, 109°   ii) sp^2, 120°   iii) sp^3, 109°

(d) i) sp^2, 120°   ii) sp^2, 120°   iii) sp^2, 120°   iv) sp^2, 120°

(e) i) sp^3, 109°   ii) sp^3, 109°   iii) sp^2, 120°   iv) sp, 180°   v) sp, 180°

(f) i) sp^3, 109°   ii) sp, 180°   iii) sp^3, 109°   iv) sp^3, 109°

So why all this focus on resonance? In general, the more stable a molecule is, the less reactive it will be. Since the delocalization of charge tends to stabilize molecules, resonance has a big impact on the reactivity of molecules.

Since it's important to recognize molecules that are stabilized by resonance, we'll next review the three basic principles of resonance delocalization.

1.   Resonance structures can never be drawn through atoms that are truly sp^3 hybridized. Remember that an sp^3-hybridized atom is one with a total of four σ bonds and/or lone electron pairs.

No resonance
structures possible!

No resonance structures are
possible with these electrons.

No resonance structures are
possible with these electrons.

2. Resonance structures usually involve electrons that are adjacent to (one atom away from) a π bond or an unhybridized *p* orbital. Here are some examples of molecules that are resonance stabilized:

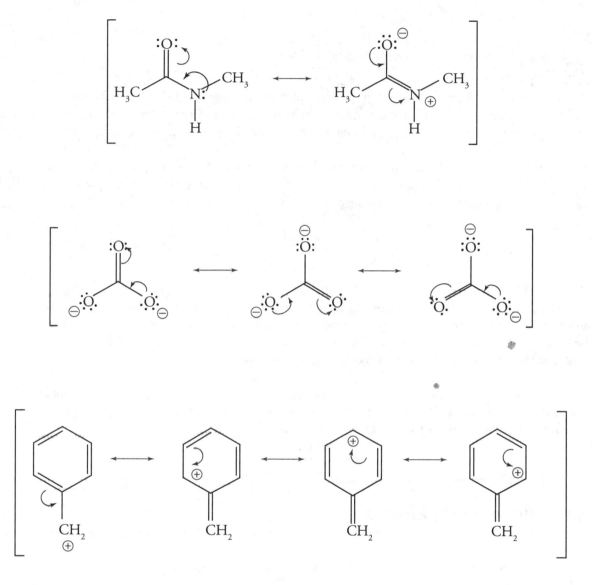

3. Resonance structures of lowest energy are the most important. Remember that the evaluation of resonance structure stability involves three main criteria:
   a. Resonance contributors in which the octet rule is satisfied for all atoms are more important than ones in which it is not. This is the most important of the three criteria listed here and takes priority over items b and c below.
   b. Resonance contributors that minimize separation of charge (formal charge) are better than those with a large separation of charge.
   c. In structures with formal charge(s), the more important resonance contributor has negative charges on the more electronegative atom(s), and positive charge(s) on the less electronegative atom(s).

Now that we can identify valid resonance structures of any given molecule and rank those resonance structures based on their relative energies, let's use this information to demonstrate the close relationship between stability and reactivity by examining acidity.

Acidity

While acids and bases will be covered in detail in Chapter 11 of the *MCAT General Chemistry Review*, we will now examine how the organic chemistry principles we've just discussed can help explain the acidity of a compound, as well as help us understand the relative acidity of several functional groups.

Firstly, let's review the definition of a Brønsted-Lowry acid. Simply put, it's a molecule that can donate a proton (H^+), and once the molecule has done so, it most commonly takes on a negative charge. This deprotonated structure is referred to as the conjugate base of the acid.

$$HCl \longrightarrow H^+ + Cl^-$$
$$\text{acid} \qquad\qquad\qquad \text{conjugate}$$
$$\text{base}$$

The strength of an acid refers to the degree to which it dissociates (or donates its proton) in solution. The more the acid dissociates, the stronger the acid is said to be. Acids that dissociate completely are said to be strong. Most organic acids, and all organic acids you're likely to see on the MCAT, are said to be weak acids because they do NOT dissociate completely in solution.

The strength of the acid is determined by the extent to which the negative charge on the conjugate base is stabilized. This means all you need to rank the relative acidity of organic compounds on the MCAT is your background in ranking the stability of reactive intermediates.

Electronegativity Effects

For example, let's compare the acidity of an alcohol like propanol and an alkane like propane. If we compare the stability of each conjugate base, we find that the alkoxide ion is a relatively stable species compared to the carbanion since the negative charge is located on the very electronegative oxygen atom rather than on a carbon atom.

$$CH_3CH_2CH_2 - \ddot{\underset{\cdot\cdot}{O}} - H$$

an alcohol

$$CH_3CH_2CH_2 - \underset{\cdot\cdot}{\overset{\cdot\cdot}{O}} \ominus$$

an alkoxide ion

$$CH_3CH_2CH_2 - H$$

an alkane

$$CH_3CH_2\overset{\cdot\cdot}{C}H_2 \ominus$$

a carbanion

Therefore, alcohols are considerably more acidic than hydrocarbons.

Resonance Effects

Let's next compare the relative acidities of propanol and propanoic acid.

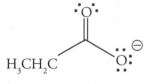

a carboxylic acid   *a carboxylate ion*

In the carboxylate ion, the electrons on the negatively charged oxygen are adjacent to a π bond and can therefore be delocalized. This leads to greater stability of the carboxylate anion and thus to higher acidity of the conjugate acid.

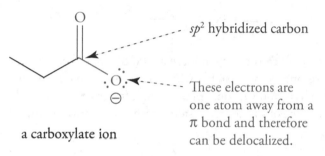

sp² hybridized carbon

These electrons are
one atom away from a
π bond and therefore
can be delocalized.

a carboxylate ion

Note that the two resonance structures of the carboxylate ion are equivalent, and are therefore of equal energy.

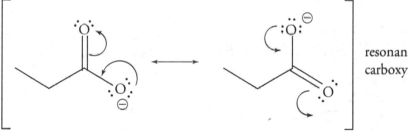

resonance structures for
carboxylate ion

In contrast, the electrons on the oxygen of the propoxide ion below have no adjacent empty *p* orbital or π system. Therefore, they are localized and highly reactive, making an alkoxide ion a very strong base (much like OH⁻) and the alcohol a weak acid.

an alkoxide ion

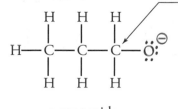

sp³ hybridized carbon

This carbon has no unhybridized
p orbital. Therefore no resonance
delocalization of the adjacent lone
pairs is possible.

n-propoxide

This makes carboxylic acids, as their name suggests, much more acidic than alcohols.

Example 4-4: Rank the following acids in order of increasing acidity:

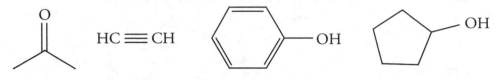

Solution: We examine the conjugate base of each acid in order to determine which one will have the more stabilized anion.

For the acetylene, there are no possible resonance structures for its conjugate base, and the negative charge is localized on carbon, an element with low electronegativity; **rank 1st** as the weakest acid.

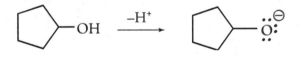

In acetone, the hydrogens next to the carbonyl are acidic because there are two resonance structures for the conjugate base of a ketone. One is stable with the negative charge on oxygen, and one is higher in energy with the negative charge on carbon. Even though it has resonance, it is less acidic than cyclopentanol (see below) because some of the charge resides on the carbon; **rank 2nd**.

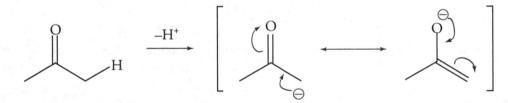

There are no possible resonance structures for this molecule, but the negative charge resides on an electronegative oxygen; **rank 3rd**.

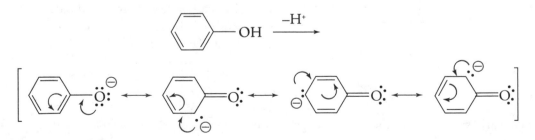

Four resonance structures are possible for the phenoxide ion because the negative charge on the oxygen is adjacent to a benzene ring. However, they are not all of equivalent energy because the negative charge resides on the less electronegative C in three of the four structures. The delocalization of charge means that a phenol (–OH group attached to a benzene ring) is more acidic than an alkyl alcohol; **rank 4th** as the strongest acid.

Note that the phenol on the previous page would still be less acidic than a carboxylic acid since both resonance structures of a carboxylate ion have the negative charge on oxygen, rather than the less electronegative carbon in the phenoxide ion.

To summarize, here is a general ranking of the relative acidities of the most important organic functional groups you are likely to see on the MCAT:

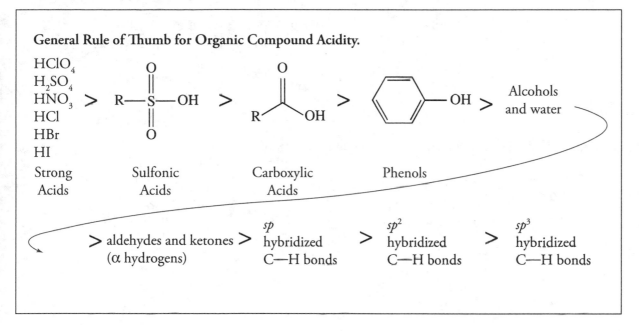

Inductive Effects

As we've just learned, the acidity of carboxylic acids compared to alcohols results from the resonance stability of the carboxylate anion. In addition, Example 4-2 briefly illustrated how electron-withdrawing substituents next to the carboxylic acid group can increase the acidity of this (or any) functional group by increasing the stability of the negative charge on the anion. To expand upon this idea, inductive effects decrease with increasing distance; the closer the electron-withdrawing group is to the acidic proton (or the negative charge on the conjugate base), the greater the stabilizing effect. The following order of acidity for the isomers of fluorobutanoic acid should help clarify this point.

Order of Acidity

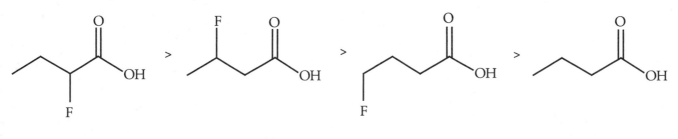

The magnitude of the effect is also dependent on the strength of the electron withdrawing substituent. In general, the more electronegative a substituent is, the greater its inductive effect will be. As shown below, while trifluoro-, trichloro-, and tribromoacetic acid all have substantially lower pK_a values than standard acetic acid (pK_a = 4.76), the trend in their acidities mirrors the electronegativity of their respective inductive group.

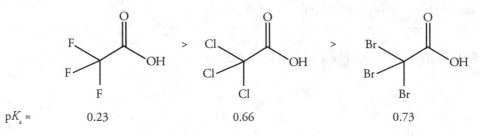

$$pK_a = \qquad 0.23 \qquad\qquad 0.66 \qquad\qquad 0.73$$

Example 4-5: Rank the following nine compounds in order of decreasing acidity.

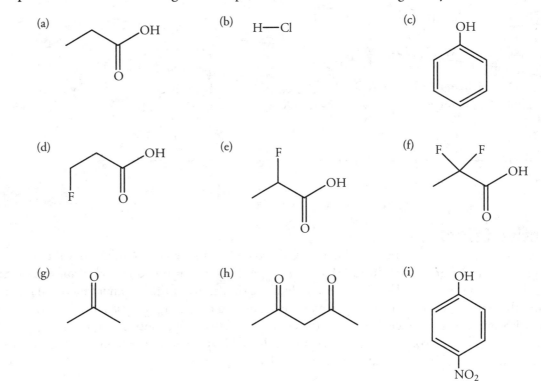

Solution:

(b) > (f) > (e) > (d) > (a)

| strong acid | difluorinated carboxylic acid | monofluorinated carboxylic acid in α position | monofluorinated carboxylic acid in β position | carboxylic acid |

> (i) > (c) ~ (h) > (g)

| phenol with electron withdrawing nitro group | phenol | diketone with 2 α protons adjacent to 2 carbonyls | ketone |

Effects of Substituents on Acidity

Electron-withdrawing substituents on phenols increase their acidity. As an example, consider *para*-nitro-phenol. The nitro group is strongly electron-withdrawing and greatly stabilizes the phenoxide ion through resonance. Once the *para*-nitrophenol is deprotonated, it's easy to see how the nitro group can withdraw electrons through the delocalized π system such that the negative charge on the phenoxide oxygen can be delocalized all the way to an oxygen atom of the nitro group. This electron-withdrawing resonance stabilization of the nitro group increases the acidity of *para*-nitrophenol as compared to a phenol that does not have electron-withdrawing substituents.

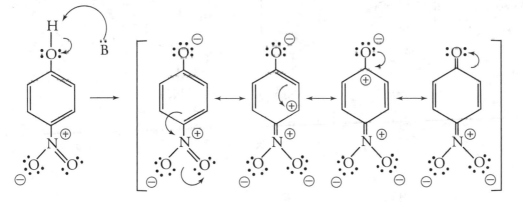

On the other hand, consider a substituted phenol that has an electron-*donating* group rather than an electron-*withdrawing* group. A good example of this is *para*-methoxyphenol. Here, it is easy to see how once *para*-methoxyphenol is deprotonated, the negative charge on the oxygen can be destabilized by the donation of a lone pair of electrons from the methoxy oxygen so a negative charge is placed on a carbon that's adjacent to the negatively charged phenoxide oxygen. Electron-donating groups tend to destabilize a phenoxide ion and decrease the acidity of substituted phenols.

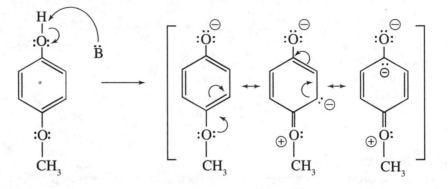

Example 4-6: For each of the following groups of three phenols, rank them in order of decreasing acidity.

(i)

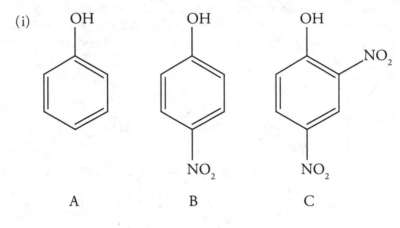

A   B   C

(ii)

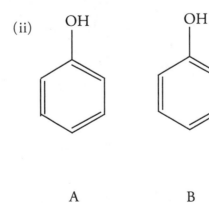
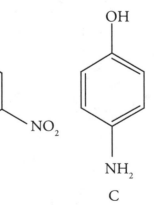

A   B   C

Solution:

(i) C > B > A. Compound C is the most acidic because of the two electron-withdrawing nitro groups. They delocalize the charge of the conjugate base, making C a stronger acid. The *para*-nitro group in B can also delocalize the charge by resonance, though not as well as the two nitro groups in choice C. Finally, A is the least acidic, since it has no electron-withdrawing groups to stabilize the charge.

(ii) B > A > C. Since the amino group in choice C is similar to the OCH_3 group discussed above due to the lone pair of electrons on the N, it is also an electron-donating group. As such, it will decrease the acidity of the phenol, making it the least acidic of the three compounds.

Nucleophiles and Electrophiles

Most organic reactions occur between nucleophiles and electrophiles. **Nucleophiles** are species that have unshared pairs of electrons or π bonds and, frequently, a negative (or partial negative, δ^-) charge. As the name *nucleophile* implies, they are "nucleus-seeking" or "nucleus-loving" molecules. Since nucleophiles are electron pair donors, they are also known as **Lewis bases**. Here are some common examples of nucleophiles:

Nucleophilicity is a measure of how "strong" a nucleophile is. There are general trends for relative nucleophilicities:

1. **Nucleophilicity increases as negative charge increases.** For example, NH_2^- is more nucleophilic than NH_3.
2. **Nucleophilicity increases going down the periodic table within a particular group.** For example, $F^- < Cl^- < Br^- < I^-$.
3. **Nucleophilicity increases going left in the periodic table across a particular period.** For example, NH_2^- is more nucleophilic than OH^-.

Trend #2 is directly related to a periodic trend introduced in general chemistry: **polarizability**. Polarizability is how easy it is for the electrons surrounding an atom to be distorted. As you go down any group in the periodic table, atoms become larger and generally more polarizable and more nucleophilic.

Trend #3 is related to the electronegativity of the nucleophilic atom. The more electronegative the atom is, the better it is able to support its negative charge. Therefore, the less electronegative an atom is, the higher its nucleophilicity.

You should note that Trend #2 should only be applied for atoms within a column of the periodic table, while Trend #3 should be applied for atoms across a row of the periodic table.

Example 4-7: In each of the following pairs of molecules, identify the one that is more nucleophilic.

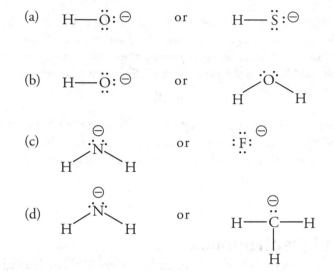

Solution:

(a) SH^-, since by Trend #2 on the previous page, S is more nucleophilic than O.
(b) OH^-, because OH^- carries a negative charge, while H_2O does not (Trend #1, previous page).
(c) NH_2^-, since F is more electronegative than N.
(d) CH_3^-, because N is more electronegative than C.

Electrophiles are electron-deficient species. They have a full or partial positive (δ^+) charge and "love electrons." Frequently, they have an incomplete octet. **Electrophilicity** is a measure of how strong an electrophile is. Since electrophiles are electron pair acceptors, they are also known as **Lewis acids**. Here are some common examples of electrophiles:

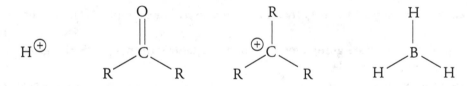

In all organic reactions (except free-radical and pericyclic reactions), nucleophiles are attracted—and donate a pair of electrons—to electrophiles. When the electrophile accepts the electron pair (a Lewis acid/Lewis base reaction), a new covalent bond forms between the two species, which we can represent symbolically like this:

$$E \overset{\oplus}{} \quad + \quad :Nu^{\ominus} \longrightarrow E\text{——}Nu$$

Leaving Groups

While students of organic chemistry often associate the discussion of leaving groups with substitution and elimination reactions, these reaction types are beyond the scope of the MCAT. However, a good understanding of leaving group ability will be useful for several reactions we'll review in Chapter 6.

Generally speaking, the biggest take-home message about leaving groups is that they are more likely to dissociate from their substrate (i.e., do their "leaving") if they are more stable in solution. Sound familiar? Our understanding of stability and reactivity is all we need to explain relative leaving group ability. For example, leaving groups that are resonance-stabilized (like tosylate, mesylate, and acetate) are some of the best ones out there. We'll discuss these groups in more detail in Chapter 6.

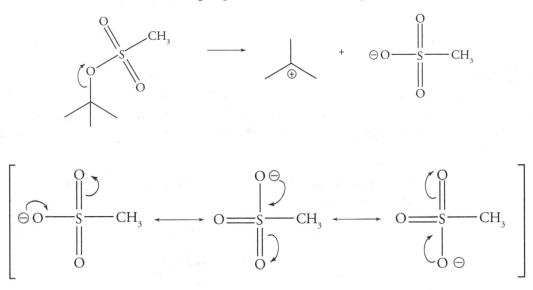

Resonance Structures of the Mesylate Leaving Group

In addition, weak bases (I⁻, Br⁻, Cl⁻, etc.) are good leaving groups because their negative charge is stabilized due to their large size. In fact, it's because basicity decreases down a family in the periodic table that leaving group ability increases. This periodic trend will be true for any family, though the halogens are the most common leaving groups you'll likely come across.

Strong bases (HO^-, RO^-, NH_2^-, etc.), on the other hand, are great electron donors because they cannot stabilize their negative charge very well, making them very reactive. As a result, these groups are more likely to stay bound to their substrate rather than dissociate in solution. As you might expect, strong bases are therefore bad leaving groups.

Now just because you're a bad leaving group one minute doesn't mean you can't be made better. For example, while the –OH group of an alcohol is unlikely to dissociate as OH⁻, treating the compound with acid protonates a lone pair of electrons on the oxygen, thereby making the –OH into $-OH_2^+$. The altered group can dissociate as a neutral water molecule, and *voila!*—no negative charge to stabilize. This trick will work for any of the strong bases listed above, and is the reason why many organic reactions are acid-catalyzed.

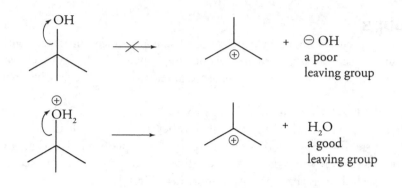

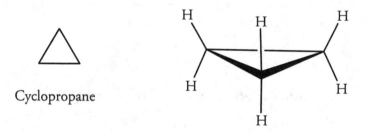

Ring Strain

The last item in our toolbox is a feature of organic molecules that, unlike inductive and resonance effects, contributes to instability in a molecule: **ring strain**. Ring strain arises when bond angles between ring atoms deviate from the ideal angle predicted by the hybridization of the atoms. Let's examine several cycloalkanes in turn.

Cyclopropane (C_3H_6) is very strained because the carbon-carbon bond angles approach 60° rather than the idealized 109° for sp^3 hybridized carbons.

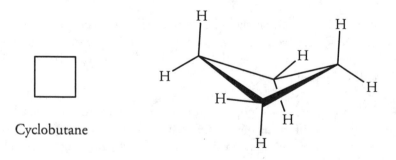

Cyclopropane

Cyclobutane (C_4H_8) might be expected to have 90° bond angles. However, one of the carbons is bent out of the plane, such that all of the bond angles are 88°. The distortion of the cyclobutane ring minimizes the eclipsing of carbon-hydrogen σ bonds on adjacent carbon atoms.

Cyclobutane

The deviation of the bond angles from the normal tetrahedral 109° causes cyclopropane and cyclobutane to be high energy compounds. The strain weakens the carbon-carbon bonds and increases reactivity of these cycloalkanes in comparison to other alkanes. For example, while it is essentially impossible to cleave the average alkane C—C single bond via hydrogenation, C—C bonds in these highly strained cyclic molecules are significantly more reactive. However, they are still much less reactive than C=C double (π) bonds.

Hydrogenation Reactions of Cyclopropane and Cyclobutane

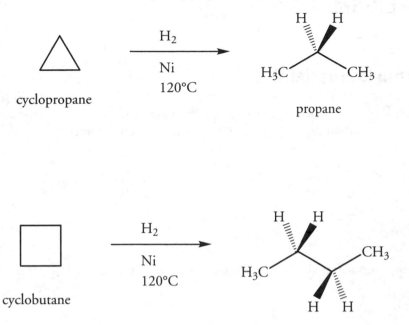

cyclopropane $\xrightarrow[\text{120°C}]{\text{H}_2 \text{ Ni}}$ propane

cyclobutane $\xrightarrow[\text{120°C}]{\text{H}_2 \text{ Ni}}$ butane

Unlike cyclopropane and cyclobutane, cyclopentane has a low degree of ring strain, and cyclohexane is strain free. Both molecules have near-tetrahedral bond angles (109°) due to the conformations they adopt. Consequently, these cycloalkanes do not undergo hydrogenation reactions under normal conditions, and react similarly to straight chain alkanes.

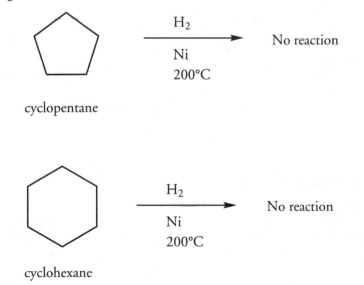

cyclopentane $\xrightarrow[\text{200°C}]{\text{H}_2 \text{ Ni}}$ No reaction

cyclohexane $\xrightarrow[\text{200°C}]{\text{H}_2 \text{ Ni}}$ No reaction

4.2 ISOMERISM

Constitutional Isomerism

Constitutional (or, less precisely, *structural*) **isomers** are compounds that have the same molecular formula but have their atoms connected together differently. Take pentane (C_5H_{12}), for example. *n*-Pentane is a fully-saturated hydrocarbon that has two additional constitutional isomers:

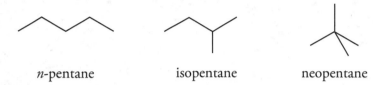

n-pentane	isopentane	neopentane

Example 4-8: Draw (and name) all the constitutional isomers of hexane, C_6H_{14}. (*Hint*: There are five of them altogether.)

Solution:

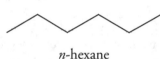 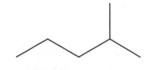 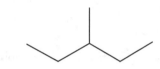

n-hexane	2-methylpentane	3-methylpentane

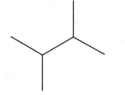 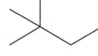 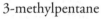

2, 3-dimethylbutane	2, 2-dimethylbutane

Conformational Isomerism

Conformational isomers are compounds that have the same molecular formula and the same atomic connectivity, but differ from one another by rotation about a σ bond. In truth, they are the exact same molecule. For saturated hydrocarbons there are two orientations of σ bonds attached to adjacent sp^3 hybridized carbons on which we will concentrate. These are the **staggered** conformation and the **eclipsed** conformation. In staggered conformations, a σ bond on one carbon bisects the angle formed by two σ bonds on the adjacent carbon. In an eclipsed conformation, a σ bond on one carbon directly lines up with a σ bond on an adjacent carbon. Both conformations can be visualized using either the flagged bond notation, or the Newman projection, as shown with ethane (C_2H_6) below.

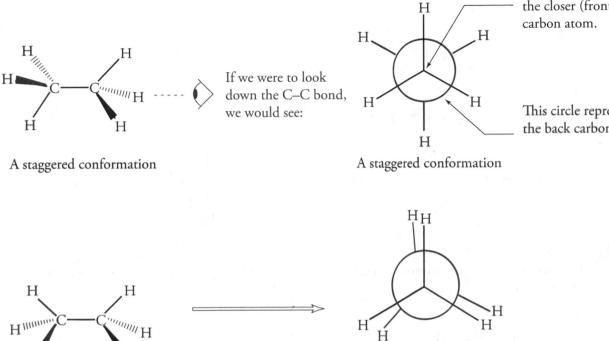

A staggered conformation

This vertex represents the closer (front) carbon atom.

A staggered conformation

This circle represents the back carbon atom.

An eclipsed conformation

An eclipsed conformation

Example 4-9: For (a) and (b), represent the flagged bond notation conformation as a Newman projection. For (c) and (d), represent the Newman projection using flagged bond notation, and be sure to label which bond you are looking down when translating from the Newman projection.

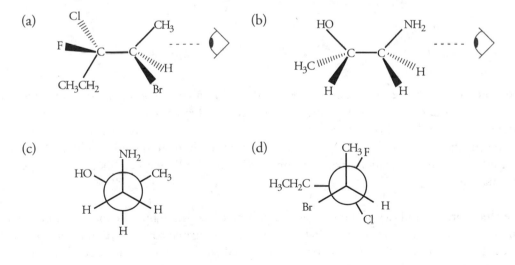

Solution:

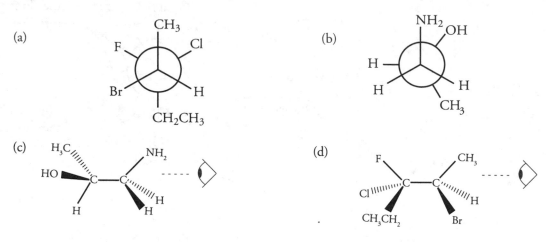

(a) (b)

(c) 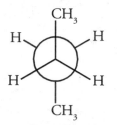 (d)

Using these notations, we turn our attention to the conformational analysis of hydrocarbons as demonstrated for *n*-butane.

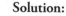

staggered conformation

less crowded
more stable

eclipsed conformation

more crowded
electronic repulsion
less stable

The σ bonds should
actually directly
line up with each other.
For clarity here,
they are not
directly aligned.

It's important to note, however, that there are an infinite number of conformations for a molecule that has free rotation around a C—C bond, and that all of these other conformations are energetically related to the staggered and eclipsed conformations on which we will concentrate. For example, relative to the carbon atom in the rear of a Newman projection, the front carbon atom could be rotated *any number of degrees*. Any change in the rotation of one carbon, relative to its adjacent neighbor, is a change in molecular conformation.

What are the relative stabilities of the staggered conformations, the eclipsed conformations, and the infinite number of conformations that are in between them? A staggered conformation is more stable than an eclipsed conformation for two reasons. First, the staggered conformation is more stable than the eclipsed conformation because of electronic repulsion. Covalent bonds repel one another simply because they are composed of (negatively charged) electrons. That being the case, the staggered conformation is more stable than the eclipsed, since in the staggered conformation, the σ bonds are as far apart as possible, while in the eclipsed conformation they are directly aligned with one another. The other major reason the staggered conformation is more stable than the eclipsed conformation is steric hindrance. It is more favorable to have atoms attached to the σ bonds in the roomier staggered conformation where they are 60° apart, rather than the eclipsed conformation where they are directly aligned with one another. There are further aspects to consider in conformational analysis. Not all staggered conformations are of equal energy. Likewise, not all eclipsed conformations are of equal energy. There are particularly stable staggered conformations and particularly unstable eclipsed conformations. The following demonstrates this by examining all staggered and eclipsed conformations for *n*-butane.

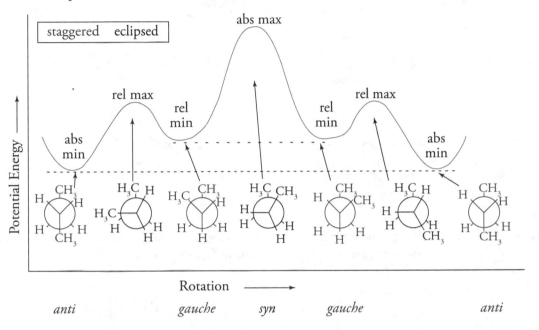

We begin our discussion with the most stable conformation of *n*-butane. This staggered conformation is referred to as the *anti* **conformation** and arises when the two largest groups attached to adjacent carbons are 180° apart. This produces the most sterically favorable, and hence the most energetically favorable (lowest energy) conformation. Now we proceed through a series of 60° rotations around the C2–C3 σ bond until we return to the initial conformation (360°). In our first rotation, we go from the *anti* staggered to an eclipsed conformation and observe the relative energy maximum that results from the alignment of the methyls and hydrogens. Next as we rotate another 60° we fall again into a staggered conformation that resides in a relative energy minimum. Notice that this energy minimum is not as low as the *anti* conformation. In this structure the methyl substituents are closer together than in the *anti* conformation. They are now 60° apart; this is referred to as a *gauche* **conformation**. A *gauche* conformation arises when the two largest groups on adjacent carbon atoms are in a staggered conformation 60° apart. In our next 60° rotation we travel to the absolute maximum on our potential energy diagram. In this eclipsed conformation, the two methyl groups are directly aligned behind one another and are therefore in the most crowded and unfavorable environment. This conformation is referred to as the *syn* **conformation**. As we continue our rotation, we fall from the absolute energy maximum and go through the corresponding staggered and eclipsed conformations encountered before.

4.2

Example 4-10: Draw a Newman projection for the most stable conformation of each of these compounds:

   (a)   2,2,5,5-tetramethylhexane (about the C3—C4 bond)
   (b)   2,2-dimethylpentane (about the C2—C3 bond)
   (c)   1,2-ethandiol

Solution:

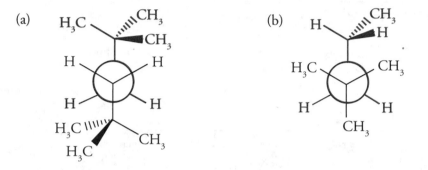

(c)   In this molecule, the *gauche* conformation is more stable than the *anti* conformation, because an intramolecular hydrogen bond can be formed in the *gauche* but not in the *anti* conformation.

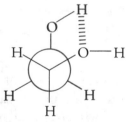

Remember that it's usually the case that the *anti* conformation is the more stable. In general, the two largest groups on adjacent carbon atoms would like to be *anti* to one another since this will minimize steric interactions. However, if the two groups are not too large and can form intramolecular hydrogen bonds with one another, then the *gauche* conformation can be more stable.

Thus far we've limited our discussion of conformational isomers to molecules with unrestricted rotation around σ bonds. Let's now consider the conformational analysis of two very common cycloalkanes, cyclopentane (C_5H_{10}) and cyclohexane (C_6H_{12}).

In cyclopentane, the pentagonal bond angle is 108° (close to normal tetrahedral of 109°), so we might expect cyclopentane to be a planar structure. If all of the carbons of cyclopentane were in a plane, however, all of the carbon-hydrogen σ bonds on adjacent carbons would eclipse each other. In order to compensate for the eclipsed C—H σ bonds, cyclopentane has one carbon out of the plane of the other carbons and so adopts a puckered conformation. This puckering allows the carbon-hydrogen σ bonds on adjacent carbons to be somewhat staggered, and thus reduces the energy of the compound. This puckered form of cyclopentane is referred to as the "envelope" form.

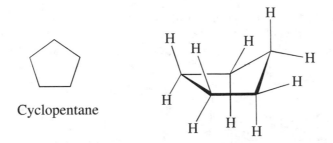

Cyclopentane

If cyclohexane were planar, it would have bond angles of 120°. This would produce considerable strain on sp^3 hybridized carbons as the ideal bond angle should be around 109°. Instead, the most stable conformation of cyclohexane is a very puckered molecule referred to as the **chair form**. In the chair conformation, four of the carbons of the ring are in a plane with one carbon above the plane and one carbon below the plane. There are two chair conformations for cyclohexane, and they easily interconvert at room temperature:

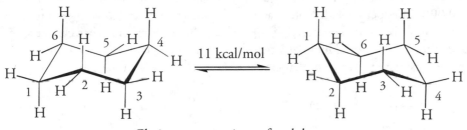

Chair representations of cyclohexane

As one chair conformation flips to the other chair conformation, it must pass through several other less stable conformations including some (referred to as *half-chair* conformations) that reside at energy maxima and one (the *twist boat* conformation) at a local energy minimum (but still of much higher energy than the chair conformations). The boat conformation represents a transition state between twist boat conformations. It is important to remember, however, that all of these conformations are much more unstable than the chair conformations and thus do not play an important role in cyclohexane chemistry.

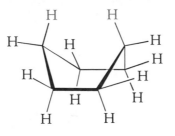

Boat conformation

Notice that there are two distinct types of hydrogens in the chair forms of cyclohexane. Six of the hydrogens lie on the equator of the ring of carbons. These hydrogens are referred to as **equatorial hydrogens**. The other six hydrogens lie above or below the ring of carbons, three above and three below; these are called **axial hydrogens**.

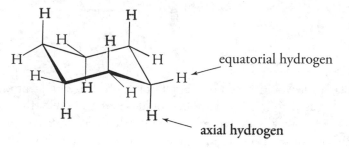

There is an energy barrier of about 11 kcal/mol between the two equivalent chair conformations of cyclohexane. At room temperature there is sufficient thermal energy to inter-convert the two chair conformations about 10,000 times per second. Note that when a hydrogen (or any substituent group) is axial in one chair conformation, it becomes equatorial when cyclohexane flips to the other chair conformation. The same is also true for an equatorial hydrogen that flips to an axial position when the chair forms interconvert. This property is demonstrated for deuterocyclohexane:

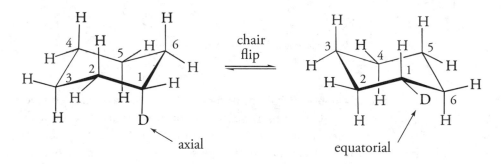

These factors become important when examining substituted cyclohexanes. Let's first consider methylcyclohexane. The methyl group can occupy either an equatorial or axial position:

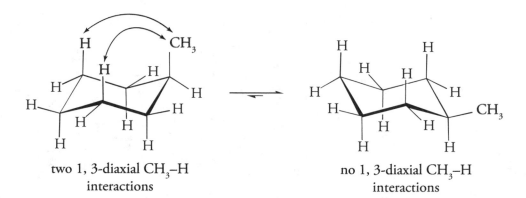

two 1, 3-diaxial CH$_3$–H
interactions

no 1, 3-diaxial CH$_3$–H
interactions

Is one conformation more stable than the other? *Yes.* It is more favorable for large groups to occupy the equatorial position rather than a crowded axial position. For a methyl group, the equatorial position is more stable by about 1.7 kcal/mol over the axial position. This is because in the axial position, the methyl group is crowded by the other two hydrogens that are also occupying axial positions on the same side of the ring. This is referred to as a **1,3-diaxial interaction**. It is more favorable for methyl to be in an equatorial position where it is pointing out, away from other atoms.

Example 4-11: In each of the following pairs of substituted cyclohexanes, identify the more stable isomer:

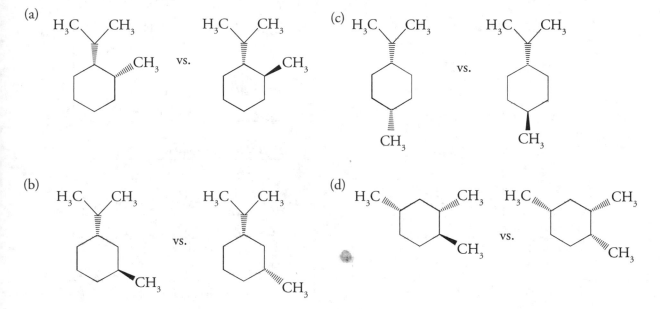

4.2

Solution: Draw chair conformations of each isomer and compare them to see which is more stable. As a good rule of thumb, it's best to first put the bulkier (i.e., the larger) substituent in a roomier equatorial position and decide if it's the more stable of the two chair conformations; it usually is. (See figures below and on the following page.)

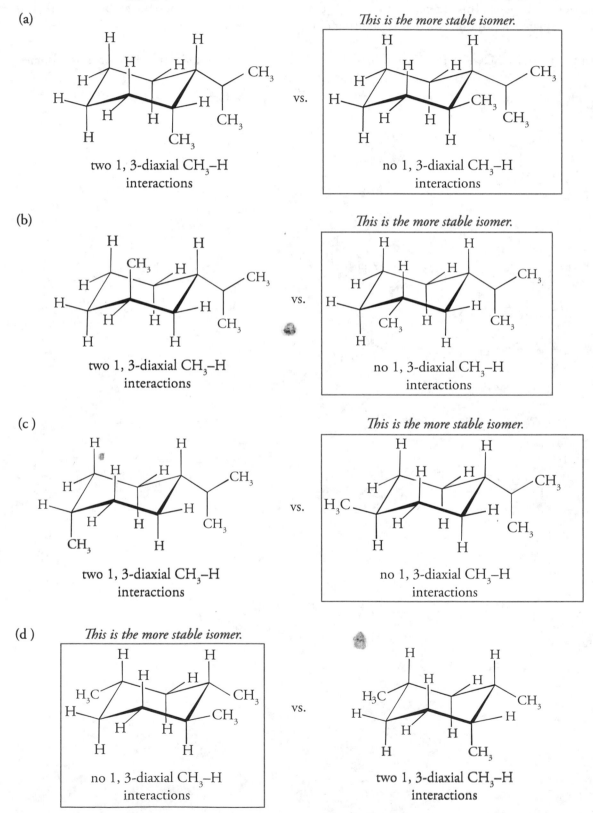

(a)

This is the more stable isomer.

two 1, 3-diaxial CH₃–H
interactions

vs.

no 1, 3-diaxial CH₃–H
interactions

(b)

This is the more stable isomer.

two 1, 3-diaxial CH₃–H
interactions

vs.

no 1, 3-diaxial CH₃–H
interactions

(c)

This is the more stable isomer.

two 1, 3-diaxial CH₃–H
interactions

vs.

no 1, 3-diaxial CH₃–H
interactions

(d)

This is the more stable isomer.

no 1, 3-diaxial CH₃–H
interactions

vs.

two 1, 3-diaxial CH₃–H
interactions

Stereoisomerism

Stereoisomerism is of major importance in organic chemistry, especially when looking at biological molecules, so several questions relating to stereochemistry routinely appear on the MCAT. **Stereoisomers** are molecules that have the same molecular formula and connectivity but differ from one another only in the spatial arrangement of the atoms. They cannot be interconverted by rotation of σ bonds. For example, consider the following two molecules:

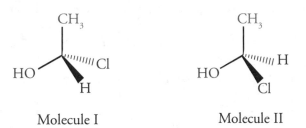

Molecule I   Molecule II

Both molecules have the same molecular formula, C_2H_5ClO, with the same atoms bonded to each other. However, if one superimposes II onto I without any rotation, the result is:

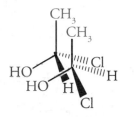

Note that while the –CH₃ and –OH groups superimpose, the –Cl and –H do not. Likewise, if we rotate Molecule II so that the –OH is pointing directly up (12 o'clock) and the –CH₃ is pointing at about 7 o'clock, and then attempt to superimpose II on I, the result is:

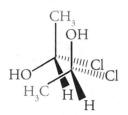

While the –Cl and the –H groups are now superimposed, the –CH₃ and the –OH are not. No matter how one rotates Molecules I and II, two of the substituent groups will be superimposed, while the other two will not. Hence they are indeed different molecules: They are stereoisomers.

4.2

Chirality

Any molecule that cannot be superimposed on its mirror image is said to be **chiral**, while a molecule that *can* be superimposed on its mirror image has a plane of symmetry and is said to be **achiral**. It's important that you be able to identify **chiral centers**. For carbon, a chiral center will have four different groups bonded to it. Note that since a carbon atom has four different groups attached to it, it must be sp^3 hybridized with (approximately) 109° bond angles and tetrahedral geometry. Such a carbon atom is also sometimes referred to as a **stereocenter**, a **stereogenic center**, or an **asymmetric center**.

Example 4-12: Identify all the chiral centers in the following molecules and determine how many possible stereoisomers each compound has by placing a star next to each chiral center. (Note: the number of possible stereoisomers equals 2^n, where n is the number of chiral centers.)

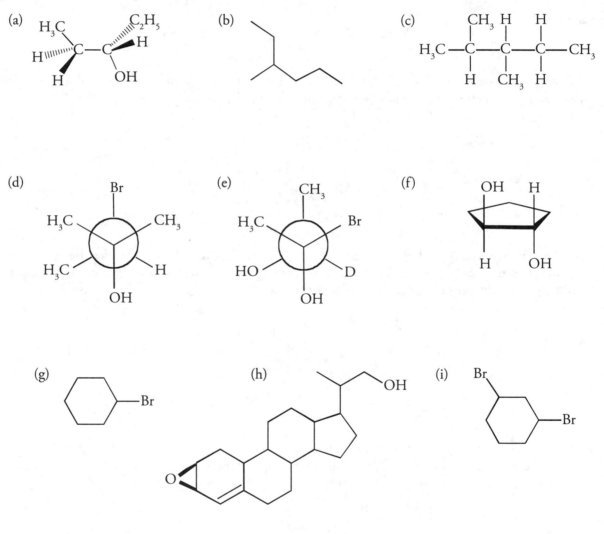

Solution:

(a)   This molecule has no chiral centers.

(b)   This molecule has 1 chiral center and, therefore, 2 possible stereoisomers:

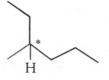

(c)   There is 1 chiral center and, therefore, 2 possible stereoisomers:

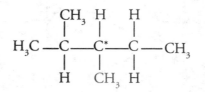

(d)   This molecule has 1 chiral center and, therefore, 2 possible stereoisomers:

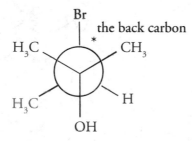

(e)   There are 2 chiral centers and, therefore, 4 possible stereoisomers:

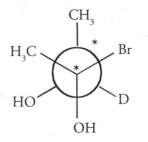

4.2

(f)   There are 2 chiral centers, which would seem to indicate 4 possible stereoisomers:

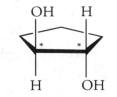

However, there are only 3, because the following "2" molecules are actually the same:

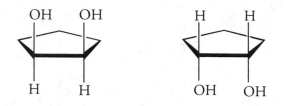

(g)   This molecule has no chiral centers.

(h)   This molecule has 9 chiral centers and, therefore, $2^9 = 512$ possible stereoisomers:

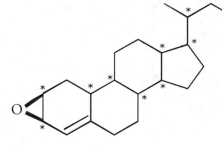

(i)   Although there are two chiral centers,

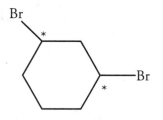

there are 3, not 4 stereoisomers, because—see (f) above—the following "two" molecules are actually the same:

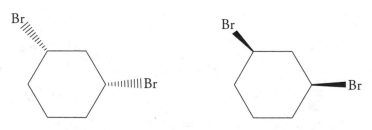

Absolute Configuration

Chiral centers (carbon atoms bearing four different substituents) can be assigned an **absolute configuration**. There is an arbitrary set of rules for assigning absolute configuration to a stereocenter (known as the Cahn-Ingold-Prelog rules), which can be illustrated using Molecule A:

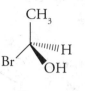

Molecule A

1. Priority is assigned to the four different substituents on the chiral center according to increasing atomic number of the atoms directly attached to the chiral center. Going one atom out from the chiral center, bromine has the highest atomic number and is given highest priority, #1; oxygen is next and is therefore #2; carbon is #3, and the hydrogen is the lowest priority group, #4:

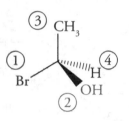

   If isotopes are present, then priority among these are assigned on the basis of atomic weight with the higher priority being assigned to the heavier isotope (since they are all of the same atomic number). For example, the isotopes of hydrogen are ^1H, ^2H = D (deuterium), and ^3H = T (tritium), and for the following molecule, we'd assign priorities as shown:

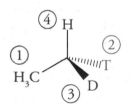

If two identical atoms are attached to a stereocenter, then the next atoms in both chains are examined until a difference is found. Once again this is done by atomic number. Note the following example:

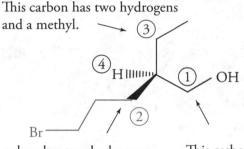

This carbon has two hydrogens and a methyl.

This carbon has two hydrogens followed by a –CH₂CH₂Br.

This carbon has two hydrogens and an –OH.

2. A multiple bond is counted as two single bonds for both of the atoms involved. For example:

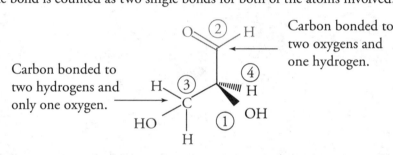

Carbon bonded to two oxygens and one hydrogen.

Carbon bonded to two hydrogens and only one oxygen.

3. Once priorities have been assigned, the molecule is rotated so that the lowest priority group points directly away from the viewer. Then simply trace a path from the highest priority group to the lowest remaining priority group. If the path traveled is *clockwise*, then the absolute configuration is **R** (from the Latin *rectus*, right). Conversely, if the path traveled is *counterclockwise*, then the absolute configuration is *S* (from the Latin *sinister*, left).

Note: The two-dimensional representation (on the left) of the following hypothetical molecule is known as the "Fischer projection," named after famous organic chemist Emil Fischer.

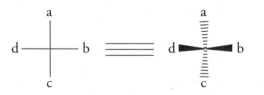

The Fischer projection is a simplification of the actual three-dimensional structure. In the Fischer projection, as shown on the right, vertical lines are assumed to go back into the page, and horizontal lines are assumed to come out of the page.

The Fischer projection will be very important in our discussion of carbohydrates and will be covered extensively in future chapters.

Example 4-13: Assign absolute configurations to the following molecules.

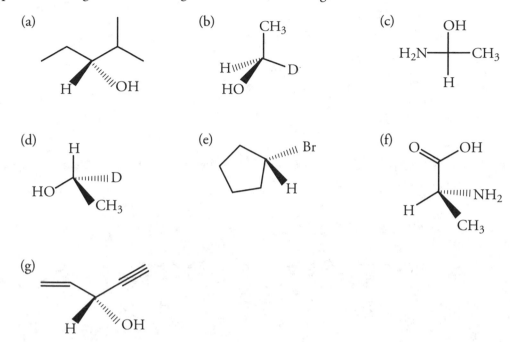

Solution:

(a)   *R.* Either rotate the molecule so the lowest priority group is in the back,

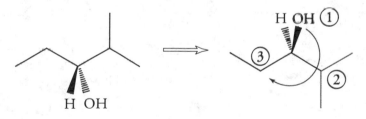

or simply trace it as it stands and invert the configuration (since the lowest priority group is coming toward you):

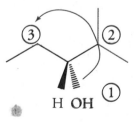

(b)   *R.* The lowest priority group is already pointing away from you and the trace is clockwise.

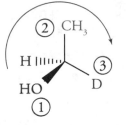

(c)   *S.* Recall Fischer notation for molecules, note that the lowest priority group is pointing away from you, and the trace is counterclockwise.

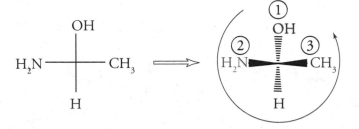

(d)   *R.* The lowest priority group is neither going into nor coming out of the plane of the page. One method is to rotate the molecule so the lowest priority group is in the back and redraw the molecule. Since the path is traveled clockwise, the configuration is *R.*

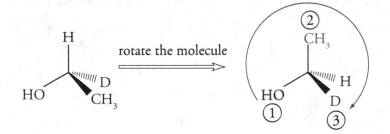

Here's a trick to help in the rotation of molecules. Exchanging two groups on a chiral center necessarily changes the absolute configuration. So in this case, it is perhaps most convenient to exchange any two groups such that the lowest priority group is going into the page:

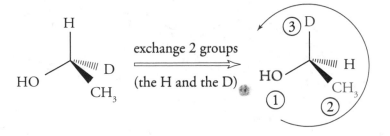

Note that this trace is going counterclockwise. Remember, however, that we exchanged two groups (the hydrogen and the deuterium), which necessarily changes the absolute configuration. Since the counterclockwise trace in the altered molecule means an *S* configuration, the true configuration is *R.*

(e)   Because this molecule is not chiral, we cannot assign it an absolute configuration.

(f)   *S*. Rotate so the lowest priority group is in back,

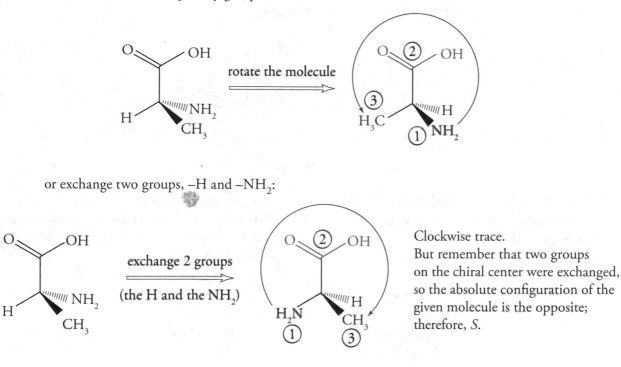

or exchange two groups, –H and –NH$_2$:

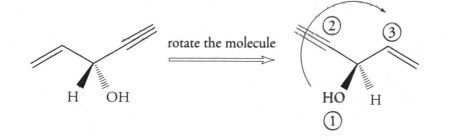

exchange 2 groups

(the H and the NH$_2$)

Clockwise trace.
But remember that two groups
on the chiral center were exchanged,
so the absolute configuration of the
given molecule is the opposite;
therefore, *S*.

(g)   *R*. Rotate so the lowest priority group is in the back:

Enantiomers

It is important to be able to identify chiral centers because, as we have seen, when there are four different groups attached to a centralized carbon, there are two distinct arrangements or configurations possible for these groups in space. Consider the following two molecules:

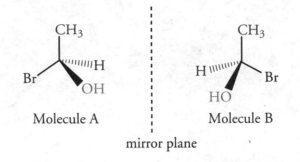

Molecule A   mirror plane   Molecule B

Molecule A has one chiral center with four different groups attached. Notice that Molecule B also has a chiral center and that the four groups attached to it are the same as those in Molecule A. Observe the mirror plane that has been drawn between Molecules A and B. Molecules A and B are mirror images of each other, but they are not superimposable; therefore, they are chiral.

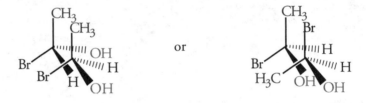

or

These molecules are **enantiomers**: non-superimposable mirror images.

Enantiomers can occur when chiral centers are present. Note that two molecules that are enantiomers will always have opposite absolute configurations; for example:

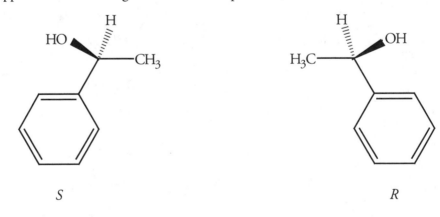

S   R

What are the properties of enantiomers? That is, how do they differ from one another? Most chemical properties such as melting point, boiling point, polarity, and solubility are the same for both pure enantiomers of an enantiomeric pair. That is, the pure enantiomers shown above will have many identical physical properties.

Optical Activity

One important property that differs between enantiomers is the manner in which they interact with plane-polarized light. A compound that rotates the plane of polarized light is said to be **optically active**. A compound that rotates plane-polarized light clockwise is said to be **dextrorotatory** (*d*), also denoted by (+), while a compound that rotates plane-polarized light in the counterclockwise direction is said to be **levorotatory** (*l*), also denoted by (–). The magnitude of rotation of plane-polarized light for any compound is called its **specific rotation**. This property is dependent on the structure of the molecule, the concentration of the sample, and the path length through which the light must travel.

A pair of enantiomers will rotate plane-polarized light with equal magnitude, but in opposite directions. For example, pure (+)-2-bromobutanoic acid has a specific rotation of +39.5°, while (–)-2-bromobutanoic acid has a specific rotation of –39.5°.

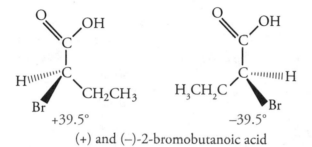

(+) and (–)-2-bromobutanoic acid

What do you think the specific rotation of an equimolar mixture of the two enantiomers above will be? Since one enantiomer will rotate plane-polarized light in one direction, while the other enantiomer will rotate light by the same magnitude in the opposite direction, the specific rotation of a 50/50 mixture of enantiomers —a **racemic mixture**—is 0°. Therefore, a racemic mixture of enantiomers, also known as a *racemate*, is not optically active.

Example 4-14: What is the specific rotation of the *R* enantiomer of 2-bromobutanoic acid? Of the *S* enantiomer?

Solution:

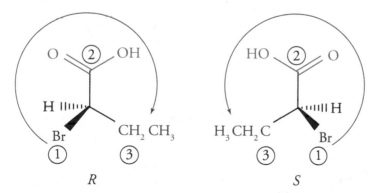

The magnitude of rotation cannot be predicted; it must be experimentally determined. It just so happens in this case that the *R* enantiomer has the (+) rotation [while the *S* enantiomer has the (–) rotation.] But be careful: **This is only coincidental. (+) and (–) say nothing about whether the absolute configuration is *R* or *S*.** There is no correlation between the sign of rotation and the absolute configuration.

4.2

Diastereomers

In the preceding discussions on stereoisomerism we have focused on molecules that have only one chiral center. What about molecules with multiple stereocenters? Remember that the number of possible stereoisomers is 2^n, where n is the number of chiral centers. If there is one chiral center, then there are two possible stereoisomers: the enantiomeric pair R and S. Two chiral centers means there are four possible stereoisomers. Consider the following molecule (3-bromobutan-2-ol), for example:

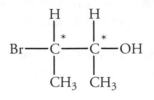

Each of the two chiral centers in 3-bromobutan-2-ol can have either R or S absolute configuration. This leads to four possible combinations of absolute configurations at the chiral centers. Both carbons could be of the S configuration or both could be of the R configuration; or, the left carbon could be R and the right carbon S, or vice versa. Here are the four possible combinations:

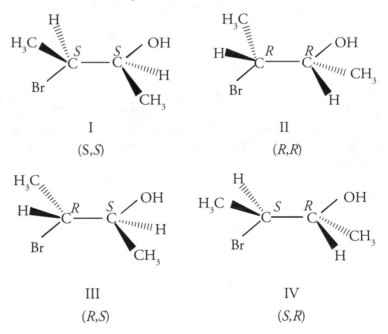

What's the relationship between Molecules I and II? Each of the two chiral centers in Molecule I is of the opposite configuration of Molecule II: S, S vs. R, R. Note that they are non-superimposable mirror images:

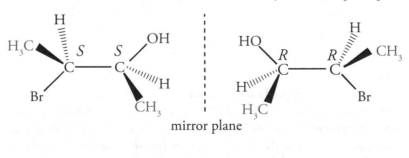

Therefore, these molecules are enantiomers. What about Molecules III and IV? Once again, each of the two chiral centers in Molecule III is of the opposite configuration of those in Molecule IV. This makes Molecules III and IV an enantiomer pair, just as we noted for Molecules I and II on the previous page. Is there a relationship between Molecules I and III?

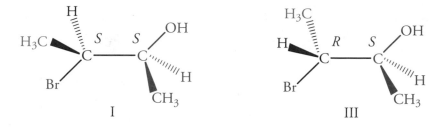

By mentally moving Molecule III to the left and aligning it over Molecule I, we see that the right chiral centers of both molecules are directly superimposable (*S* superimposes onto *S*). Also note that no matter what we do, we cannot get the left chiral centers of Molecules I and III to superimpose (*S* does not super-impose onto *R*).

Molecules I and III are diastereomers. **Diastereomers** are stereoisomers that are not enantiomers. That is, diastereomers are stereoisomers that are non-superimposable, non-mirror images. The same is true for Molecules I and IV. One of the chiral centers is of the same absolute configuration, while the other chiral center is of the opposite configuration:

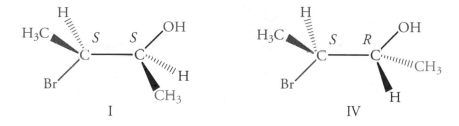

The figure below summarizes all possible stereochemical relationships between isomers containing two stereocenters. Inverting at least one, but not all, of the chiral centers within a molecule will form a diaste-reomer of that molecule. Enantiomers can be formed by inverting every stereocenter within the molecule.

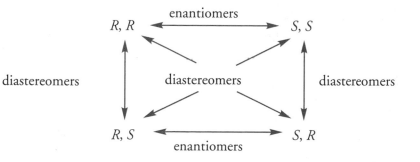

Example 4-15: For each pair of molecules below, state the relationship between them.

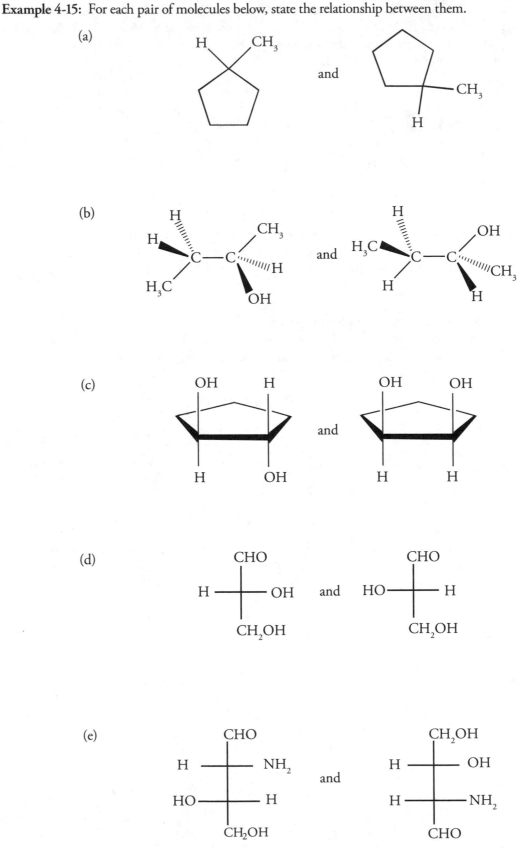

(a)

and

(b)

and

(c)

and

(d)

CHO and CHO

(e)

CHO and CH₂OH

Solution:

(a) The molecules are superimposable and therefore *identical*.

(b) The molecules are *identical*. (The left carbon is not a chiral center.)

(c) *Diastereomers.*

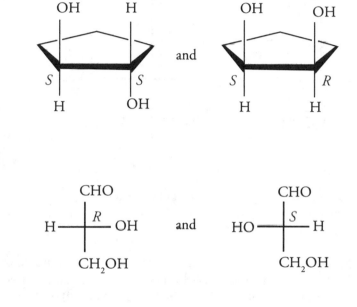

(d) *Enantiomers.*

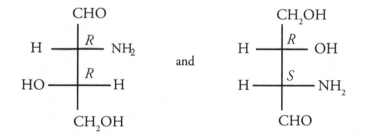

(e) *Diastereomers.*

While the structures of diastereomers are similar, their physical and chemical properties can vary dramatically. They can have different melting points, boiling points, solubilities, dipole moments, specific rotations, etc. Most importantly for the MCAT, the specific rotation of diastereomers is also different, but *there is no relationship between the specific rotations of diastereomers as there is for enantiomers*. There is no way to predict the specific rotation of one diastereomer if you know the degree of rotation of another.

Resolution of Enantiomers

Nature has evolved intricate mechanisms for the bio-synthesis of enantiomerically pure, optically active compounds. For example, L-(+)-tartaric acid, D-(+)-fructose, and L-(+)-valine are all isolated as a single enantiomer from their respective biological sources.

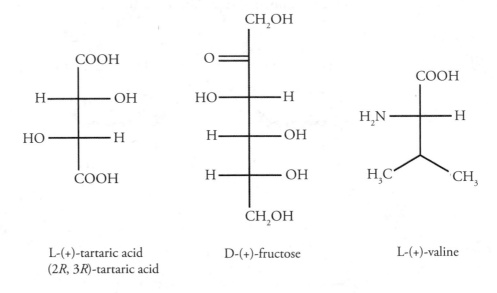

| L-(+)-tartaric acid | D-(+)-fructose | L-(+)-valine |
| (2R, 3R)-tartaric acid | | |

Unfortunately, the laboratory syntheses of enantiomerically pure compounds is often laborious and expensive. It is generally more time- and cost-effective to synthesize chiral targets as racemic mixtures. For example, the reduction of 2-butanone (achiral) to 2-butanol (chiral) yields both enantiomers.

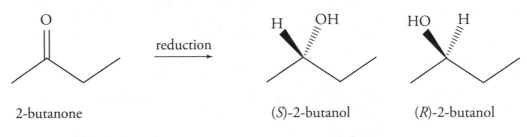

2-butanone   (S)-2-butanol   (R)-2-butanol

If only one enantiomer of 2-butanol is needed, the two alcohols must be separated. Since enantiomers have identical chemical and physical properties, separating a racemic mixture is a nontrivial process called **resolution**.

The traditional method for resolving a racemic mixture is through the use of an enantiomerically pure chiral probe, or resolving agent, that associates with the components of the mixture through either covalent bonds or intermolecular forces (like hydrogen bonds or salt interactions). The resulting products will be diastereomers, capable of separation due to their different physical properties.

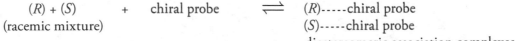

$(R) + (S)$ +   chiral probe $\rightleftharpoons$ (R)-----chiral probe
(racemic mixture) (S)-----chiral probe
                   diastereomeric association complexes

For example, racemic (±)-2-amino-2-phenylacetic acid can be resolved with enantiomerically pure (1*R*,4*R*)-(+)-10-camphorsulfonic acid, as shown in the figure below.

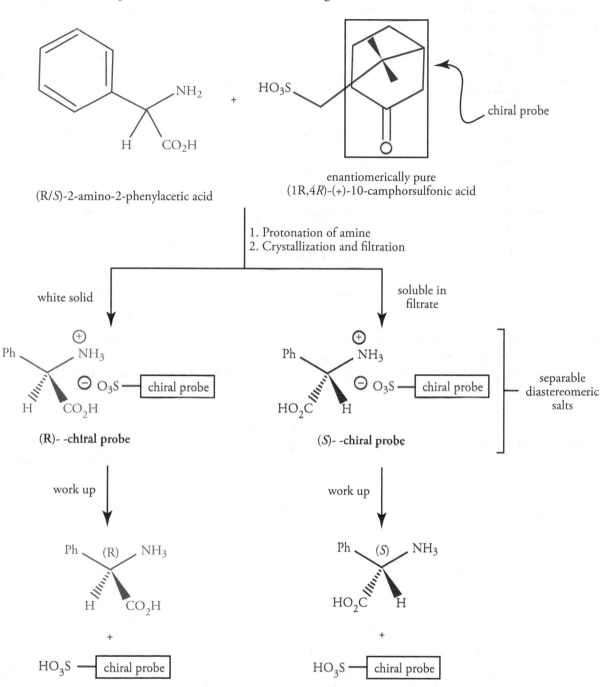

Protonation of the amine by the sulfonic acid produces two diastereomeric salts with different chemical and physical properties. In this particular instance, these salts have different solubilities; the *R* salt precipitates as a crystalline solid while the *S* salt remains dissolved in the filtrate. A simple filtration process is used to separate the two, which can be released from the probe and isolated as enantiomerically pure material in a subsequent work-up step.

4.2

Epimers

Epimers are a subclass of diastereomers that differ in their absolute configuration at a single chiral center (only *one* stereocenter is inverted). To illustrate epimeric relationships, let's look at the Fischer projections of some sugars (see Chapter 7):

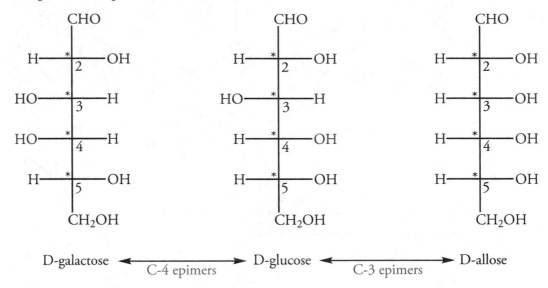

The prefix D on the name of these molecules refers to the orientation of the hydroxyl group (–OH) on the highest-numbered chiral center in a Fischer projection (C-5 in these cases). When the hydroxyl group is on the *right* of this carbon in the Fischer projection, the molecule is a D sugar. (When the hydroxyl group is on the *left*, the molecule is an L sugar.)

You must understand that D and L, like *R* and *S*, are entirely unrelated to optical activity, (+) or (–). Distinctions between D and L (or between *R* and *S*) can be made just by looking at a drawing of the molecule, but distinctions between (+) and (–) can be made only by running experiments in a polarimeter.

- *R* or *S* = absolute configuration (structure)
- D or L = relative configuration (structure)
- (+) or (–) = observed optical rotation (property)

Concerning the three sugars above, we see that D-glucose and D-galactose differ in stereochemistry at only one chiral center (C-4). Thus, D-glucose and D-galactose are said to be C-4 epimers, and C-4 is called the **epimeric carbon**. Likewise, D-glucose and D-allose differ in structure at a single chiral center (C-3). D-Glucose and D-allose are C-3 epimers, with C-3 being the epimeric carbon.

What about D-galactose and D-allose? What is the relationship between these two molecules? We can see that these two sugars differ at two chiral centers (C-3 and C-4). At least one, but not all, of the stereocenters have been inverted. Therefore they are diastereomers, but *NOT* epimers. Note that all epimers are diastereomers, but not all diastereomers are epimers.

Anomers

Epimers that form as a result of ring closure are known as **anomers**. For the MCAT, anomers will be encountered only with regard to sugar chemistry. To illustrate anomerism, consider D-glucose. Open-chain glucose exists in equilibrium with cyclic glucose, known as *glucopyranose*. Cyclization occurs when the C-5 hydroxyl group attacks the carbonyl (C=O) carbon, C-1. This converts a carbon with three substituents to a carbon with four different substituents. Thus, a new stereocenter is formed (C-1), and it can assume one of two possible forms: with the hydroxyl group *down*, it is α; with the hydroxyl group *up*, it is β. It is the orientation at C-1 that distinguishes the two anomers, and C-1 is known as the **anomeric center** (or **anomeric carbon**).

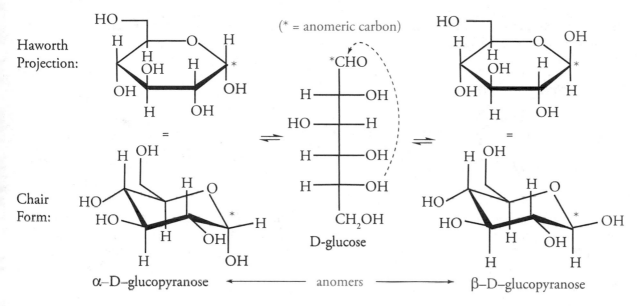

Meso Compounds

Let's look at another molecule with more than one stereocenter. Consider 2,3-butanediol:

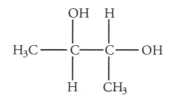

Upon inspection, we determine that there are two chiral centers and therefore four possible stereoisomers. Notice that both chiral centers have the same groups attached to them: –H, –CH$_3$, –OH, and –CH(OH) CH$_3$. When the same four groups are attached to two chiral centers, the molecule can have an internal plane of symmetry. Let's examine this a little more closely. We first consider the *R, R* stereoisomer and the *S, S* stereoisomer of 2,3-butanediol:

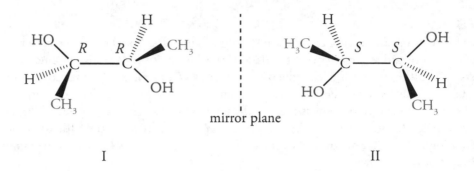

I   II

There are two things to notice here. First, I and II are non-superimposable mirror images and therefore enantiomers. Second, in both I and II there is no internal plane of symmetry. This is demonstrated for Molecule II:

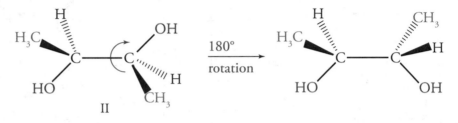

The –OH groups line up on the two chiral centers, but the –CH₃ groups and –H atoms do not. The optical rotation of a 50/50 mixture of molecules I and II would measure zero because this is a racemic mixture.

Now look at the R, S stereoisomer and its mirror image:

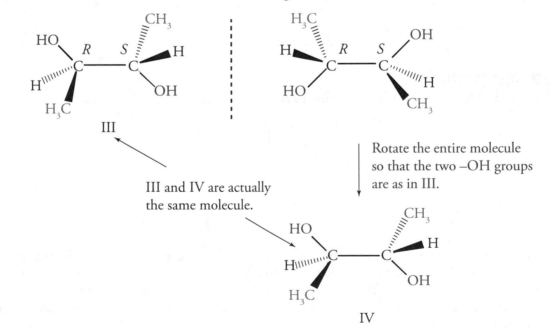

It turns out that Molecules III and IV are directly superimposable and therefore identical. This is because there is an internal plane of symmetry within the molecule.

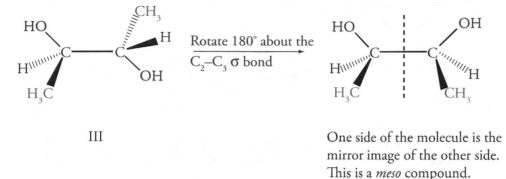

Rotate 180° about the
C_2–C_3 σ bond

III

One side of the molecule is the mirror image of the other side. This is a *meso* compound.

When there's an internal plane of symmetry in a molecule that contains chiral centers, the compound is called a **meso** compound. Actually then, 2,3-butanediol has only *three* stereoisomers, not four. Molecules I and II are enantiomers, while III and IV are the same molecule. Molecule III (or IV) is an example of a meso compound. Meso compounds have chiral centers but are not optically active (so they are achiral) because one side of the molecule is a mirror image of the other. In a sense, the optical activity imparted by one side of the molecule is canceled by its other side.

Example 4-16: Which of the following molecules are optically active?

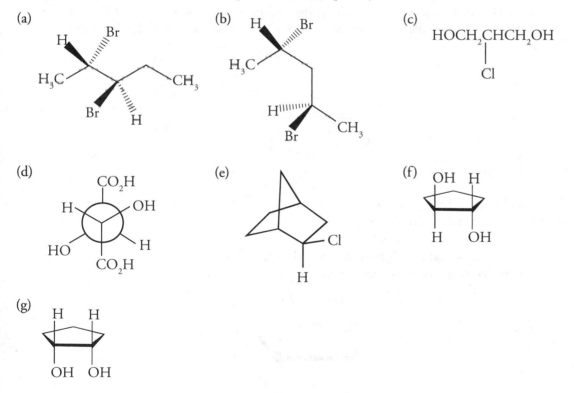

(c)

HOCH$_2$CHCH$_2$OH
|
Cl

4.2

Solution:

(a)   This molecule is optically active. It has two chiral centers, but no internal mirror plane. Therefore it is not a meso compound and will rotate plane-polarized light.

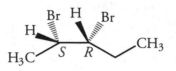

(b)   This molecule is a meso compound due to its two chiral centers and internal mirror plane. It will be optically inactive. Be sure to look for rotations around σ bonds in order to find the mirror planes of some molecules.

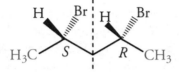

(c)   This molecule has no chiral centers, so will have no optical activity.

(d)   By rotating around the C-2 to C-3 bond to put the molecule into an eclipsed conformation, you can see that there is an internal mirror plane in the molecule. Since C-2 and C-3 are also chiral centers with four different substituents, this is a meso compound, and will be optically inactive.

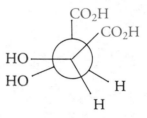

(e)   This molecule has three chiral centers (the two bridgehead carbons are chiral), but no plane of symmetry. It is therefore chiral and optically active.

(f)   There is no mirror image in this molecule even though it has two chiral centers (they have the same absolute configuration). It will therefore be optically active.

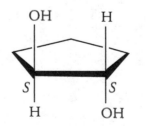

(g) This molecule does have an internal mirror plane, and its two chiral centers have opposite absolute configurations. It is therefore meso, and not optically active.

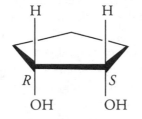

Geometric Isomers

Geometric isomers are diastereomers that differ in orientation of substituents around a ring or a double bond. Cyclic hydrocarbons and double bonds (alkenes) are constrained by their geometry, meaning they do not rotate freely about all bonds. So, there's a difference between having substituents on the same side of the ring (or double bond) and having substituents on opposite sides. For example, the following are geometric isomers of 1,2-dimethylcyclohexane:

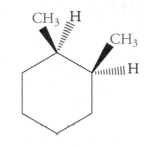
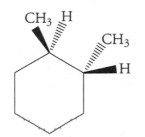

cis-1,2-dimethylcyclohexane   *trans*-1,2-dimethylcyclohexane

Priority of substituent groups is assigned the same way as for absolute configuration. On C-1, the methyl group is given higher priority than the H, and the same is true on C-2. The molecule in which the two higher-priority groups are on the same side is termed *cis*, and the molecule in which the two higher-priority groups are on opposite sides of the ring is termed *trans*.

The same-side/opposite-side substituent relativity also occurs with double bonds, but in this case the stereochemistry is officially designated by (*Z*) or (*E*). The (*Z*)/(*E*) notation is a completely unambiguous way to specify the appropriate stereochemistry at the double bond. In this system, a high and low priority group are assigned at each carbon of the double bond based on atomic number, just as with absolute configuration. If the two high priority groups are on the *same* side, the configuration at the double bond is *Z* (from the German *zusammen*, meaning *together*). On the other hand, if the two high priority groups are on opposite sides of the double bond, the configuration is referred to as *E* (from the German *entgegen*, meaning *opposite*). Be aware, that the MCAT may also use the terms *cis* and *trans* when referring to double bonds. However, this is usually reserved for the case when there is one H attached to each carbon of the double bond, as shown below. The geometric isomers of 2-bromo-1-chloropropene and of 1,2-dibromoethene are shown below:

Highest priority groups (Br and Cl) on same side, so *Z*.

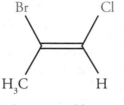

Highest priority groups (Br and Cl) on opposite side, so *E*.

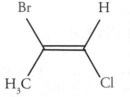

(*Z*)-2-bromo-1-chloropropene

(*E*)-2-bromo-1-chloropropene

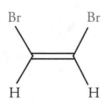

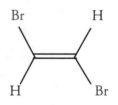

cis-1,2-dibromoethene

trans-1,2-dibromoethene

SUMMARY OF ISOMERS

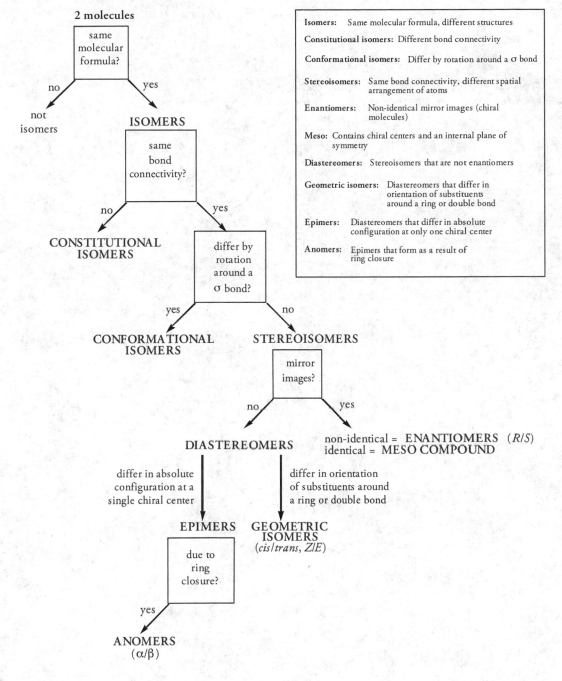

Isomers: Same molecular formula, different structures

Constitutional isomers: Different bond connectivity

Conformational isomers: Differ by rotation around a σ bond

Stereoisomers: Same bond connectivity, different spatial arrangement of atoms

Enantiomers: Non-identical mirror images (chiral molecules)

Meso: Contains chiral centers and an internal plane of symmetry

Diastereomers: Stereoisomers that are not enantiomers

Geometric isomers: Diastereomers that differ in orientation of substituents around a ring or double bond

Epimers: Diastereomers that differ in absolute configuration at only one chiral center

Anomers: Epimers that form as a result of ring closure

Chapter 4 Summary

- Saturated compounds have the general formula C_nH_{2n+2}; unsaturated molecules contain rings or π bonds.

- As the substitution of carbocations increases, so does their stability due to the inductive effect; carbanions are more stable when they are less substituted.

- Resonance stabilization results from the ability of π electrons or charge to move and delocalize through a system of conjugated π bonds or unhybridized p orbitals.

- Brønsted-Lowry acids are proton donors, and are stronger (dissociate more) when their conjugate bases are most stable in solution.

- Acidity of carboxylic acids results from the resonance stability of the carboxylate anion.

- Electron-withdrawing groups increase the acidity of carboxylic acids by stabilizing the negative charge of the carboxylate anion via the inductive effect.

- Nucleophiles are Lewis bases and are electron rich, while electrophiles are Lewis acids and are electron deficient.

- Nucleophiles are stronger when negatively charged, less electronegative, or larger in size.

- Leaving groups are more likely to leave as their stability in solution increases (uncharged and/or larger groups are usually better LGs).

- Compounds with the same molecular formula are known as *isomers*; structural, or constitutional isomers differ by the connectivity of atoms in the molecule.

- Conformational isomers differ by rotation around a σ bond.

- Stereoisomers have the same atom connectivity, but different spatial orientation of atoms.

- Chiral molecules have chiral centers (carbon with four different substituents), are not superimposable on their mirror image, and rotate plane-polarized light.

- Enantiomers are non-superimposable mirror images and have opposite absolute configuration at all chiral centers.

- Enantiomers rotate plane-polarized light an equal magnitude, but in opposite direction, therefore a 50:50 mixture of enantiomers, or a racemic mixture, is not optically active.

- The process of separating a mixture of enantiomers is called resolution, and entails conversion of the racemic mixture into a pair of separable diastereomers temporarily before converting back to the pure, chiral enantiomers.

- Diastereomers are stereoisomers that are not mirror images; they differ in absolute configuration for at least one, but not all carbons.

- Epimers are diastereomers that differ in absolute configuration at only one stereocenter.

- Geometric isomers are diastereomers that are *cis/trans* (or *Z/E*) pairs on a ring or double bond. When highest priority groups are on the same side of a ring or bond the molecule is *cis* (or *Z*); when they're on opposite sides, the compound is *trans* (or *E*).

- Meso compounds are achiral molecules with chiral centers and an internal mirror plane.

CHAPTER 4 FREESTANDING PRACTICE QUESTIONS

1. In the molecule below, what are the hybridizations of C_1, C_2, C_3, and C_4 respectively?

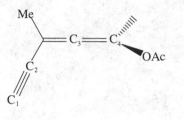

A) sp, sp, sp^2, sp^2
B) sp, sp, sp, sp^2
C) sp^2, sp^2, sp, sp
D) sp^2, sp, sp, sp

2. Which of the following structures represents the most stable possible resonance structure for acetic acid (CH_3CO_2H)?

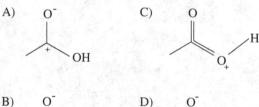

3. Rank the conformations of 2-aminoethanol by increasing stability.

A) *anti* < *gauche* < eclipsed
B) eclipsed < *anti* < *gauche*
C) *gauche* < *anti* < eclipsed
D) eclipsed < *gauche* < *anti*

4. The most stable conformation of the following substituted cyclohexane has the methyl groups in which of the following positions?

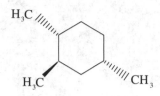

A) 2 Equatorial and 1 axial
B) All axial
C) All equatorial
D) 2 Axial and 1 equatorial

5. How many stereoisomers are possible for cortisone acetate (shown below)?

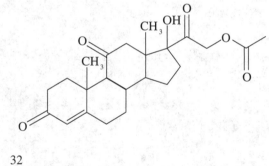

A) 32
B) 64
C) 128
D) 256

6. What is the correct IUPAC name for the following molecule?

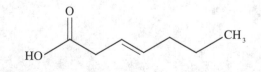

A) (*E*)-3-heptenoic acid
B) (*E*)-4-heptenoic acid
C) (*Z*)-3-heptenoic acid
D) (*Z*)-4-heptenoic acid

7. Which of the following is the strongest nucleophile?

A) CN^-
B) OH^-
C) CH_3OH
D) NH_3

8. Which of the following lists two pairs of diastereomers?

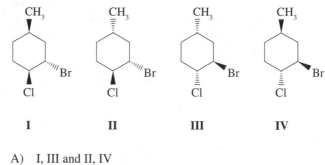

I   II   III   IV

A) I, III and II, IV
B) I, II and II, III
C) I, III and I, IV
D) II, IV and III, IV

CHAPTER 4 PRACTICE PASSAGE

In mammalian systems, aromatic hydrocarbons are enzymatically metabolized by cytochrome P_{450} into arene oxides when ingested or inhaled. Arene oxides are compounds in which one of the double bonds of an aromatic ring has been converted into an epoxide. These molecules can rearrange to form phenols, which are harmlessly excreted. As shown in Figure 1, arene oxide rearrangement requires the formation of an intermediate carbocation and subsequent hydride shift.

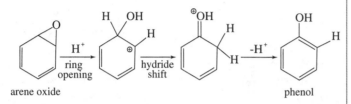

Figure 1 Arene oxide rearrangement

Benzo[a]pyrene, found in tobacco smoke and automobile exhaust, is one of the most troublesome natural arene oxides because it is a procarcinogen due to its bioconversion to a number of harmful molecules such as the 7,8-diol epoxide shown in Figure 2. The danger of the 7,8-diol epoxide lies in the unwillingness of the epoxide ring to rearrange and form a phenol. Instead, the diol epoxide intercalates in DNA and is covalently bound by 2′-deoxyguanosine nucleosides, leading to point mutations in the course of DNA replication.

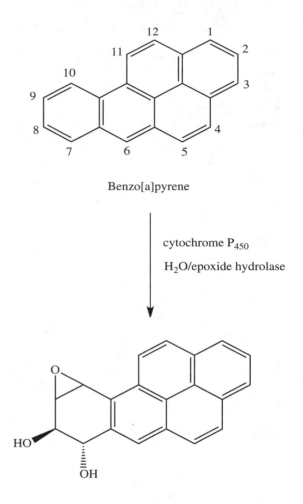

Benzo[a]pyrene

Benzo[a]pyrene-7,8-dihydrodiol-9,10-epoxide

Figure 2 Oxidation of Benzo[a]pyrene

1. Determine the absolute configurations of Carbons 7 and 8 of the diol epoxide shown in Figure 2.

A) 7R, 8R
B) 7R, 8S
C) 7S, 8S
D) 7S, 8R

2. All of the following statements about the diol epoxide shown in Figure 2 are correct EXCEPT:

A) the epoxide bears the same type of leaving group as an ether.
B) ring strain and torsional strain increase the free energy of the epoxide.
C) the epoxide may react under strongly acidic conditions.
D) the epoxide oxygen atom is capable of donating a hydrogen bond.

3. Rank the following four substances in order of increasing reactivity with an arene oxide.

   I.   Hydroxide
   II. Ammonia
   III. Methide
   IV. Water

A) III < I < II < IV
B) IV < II < I < III
C) IV < II < III < I
D) II < IV < I < III

4. Which labeled atom of the nucleoside shown below is responsible for intercalation of the diol epoxide?

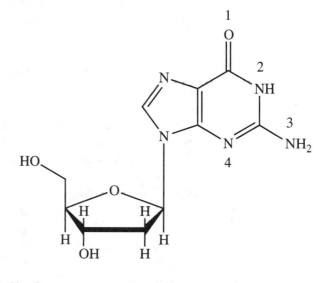

A) 1
B) 2
C) 3
D) 4

5. Which of the following arene oxides will react as in Figure 1 to form the most stable carbocation intermediate?

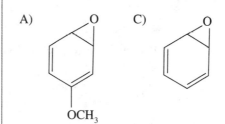

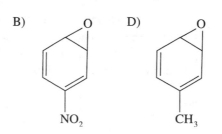

SOLUTIONS TO CHAPTER 4 FREESTANDING PRACTICE QUESTIONS

1. **B** Both C_1 and C_2 make up the triple bond. They are both *sp* hybridized so you can eliminate choices C and D. C_3 is part of an allene. The bonds that it forms with its neighbors are linear (180°), so it is also *sp*. You can eliminate choice A, which leaves choice B as the correct choice. C_4 has a double bond and two single bonds so it is *sp²*.

2. **B** Good resonance structures must do the following: obey the octet rule, accrue the fewest charges possible, and place negative charges on electronegative atoms and positive charges on electropositive atoms (listed in priority). Further, resonance structures don't represent oxidation or reduction of molecules, and as such the total charge of each structure must be the charge of the molecule. This eliminates choices C and D. Choices A and B are both valid resonance structures, but only choice B places a full octet on all non-H atoms.

3. **B** Since this is a ranking question, look for obvious extremes and eliminate answers. Choices A and C should be eliminated because the eclipsed conformation is always the least stable due to sterics and electron repulsions in aligned bonds. Choice D is the more enticing answer of the remaining two because the general rule of thumb is that the *anti* conformation is the most stable because the bulky groups are farthest apart, while they are 60° apart in a *gauche* conformation. This question is tricky, however, because in this case there is intramolecular hydrogen bonding which can occur in the *gauche* conformation, making it the most stable one (eliminate choice D).

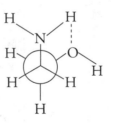

4. **A** Choice B can be eliminated before analyzing the structure since if all three substituents could be axial, then by a ring flip, all three could also be equatorial. The more stable chair conformation puts substituents in an equatorial position since they are less sterically crowded than those in axial positions. Similarly, if choice A is true of the molecule, then by ring flip, choice D must be also. Therefore choice D should be eliminated since it has more axial substituents. Between choices A and C, only choice A fits the compound shown because the relationship between the methyl groups on Carbons 1 and 2 is *trans* and the relationship between the methyl groups on Carbons 1 and 4 is *cis*. In this conformation, the methyl groups on Carbons 1 and 2 would be found in the equatorial position and the methyl group on Carbon 4 would be axial, making A the better choice.

5. **B** The maximum number of stereoisomers is given by the formula 2^n, where *n* equals the number of stereocenters. Cortisone acetate has six stereocenters and $2^6 = 64$. Five of the six ring junctures are chiral centers (all *sp³* carbons), as is the carbon with the OH substituent. Choice A would correspond to five stereocenters, choice C would require seven stereocenters, and choice D would correspond to a compound with eight stereocenters.

6. **A** When naming a compound, number the carbons starting at the end nearest a functional group (the carboxylic acid in this case). Based on the position of the double bond in the molecule, you can eliminate choices B and D. Since the two largest substituents on each carbon of the double bond are on opposite sides of the bond, the double bond has E stereochemistry; therefore, eliminate choice C.

7. **A** Nucleophiles are electron rich. While neutral compounds that have lone pairs can be nucleophilic, negatively charged nucleophiles tend to be stronger (eliminate choices C and D). The stronger nucleophile is the more reactive nucleophile; more reactive corresponds to less stable. Therefore, the nucleophile that is less able to stabilize a negative charge will be the stronger nucleophile. For choices A and B, the negative charge resides on the C and O, respectively. Since carbon is less electronegative than oxygen, it is therefore less able to stabilize a negative charge, making cyanide the best nucleophile (eliminate choice B).

8. **B** Stereoisomers in which all stereocenters are inverted are enantiomers, while stereoisomers with at least one, but not all, inverted chiral centers are diastereomers. Molecules I and III are an enantiomeric pair (eliminate choices A and C); Molecules II and IV are enantiomers as well (eliminate choice D). All other pairs of molecules are diastereomers.

SOLUTIONS TO CHAPTER 4 PRACTICE PASSAGE

1. **D**

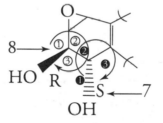

Note that the configuration for Carbon 7 reads as R, but because the hydroxyl group occupies an into-plane position, this assignment is incorrect. One way to get around this is to exchange the hydroxyl group's position with the hydrogen also on this carbon. Doing so will place the hydroxyl group in a correct position, which results in a clockwise trace. This reads as R but because two groups have been exchanged, the true configuration is S. Once the configuration of Carbon 7 is determined to be S, choices A and B can be eliminated.

2. **D** Epoxides and ethers all bear an OR leaving group so choice A can be eliminated. Choice B is incorrect because epoxides, due to their 3-point ring structure, possess ring strain and torsional strain, which imparts a relatively high free energy. Under acidic conditions, the epoxide oxygen atom will be protonated, which permits a nucleophile to perform an S_N2 reaction, also eliminating choice C. Choice D is the only answer choice consistent with the EXCEPT wording of the question because epoxides are only capable of accepting hydrogen bonds, not donating them.

3. **B** Each of the four substances listed will act as nucleophiles with an arene oxide. The strongest nucleophile has a negative charge on the least electronegative atom, which is carbon. Choices B and D both list methide as the strongest nucleophile (eliminate choices A and C). The weakest nucleophile is going to be listed first. The choice is between water and ammonia. Since nitrogen is less electronegative than oxygen, NH_3 is a stronger nucleophile than water (eliminate choice D).

4. **C** As stated in the passage, intercalation of the 2'-deoxyguanosine nucleoside occurs via a co-valent bond with the diol epoxide. As all labeled atoms in the molecule shown contain a lone pair of electrons, this suggests that the 2'-deoxyguanosine nucleoside can act as a nucleophile. The site that is most nucleophilic will therefore be the site most likely to react. O-1 is unlikely to react, as oxygen is not as electron-donating as the three remaining nitro-gen-based choices (eliminate choice A). N-2 is an amide nitrogen engaged in resonance with the adjacent carbonyl, decreasing its ability to donate electrons (eliminate choice B). The lone pairs available on N-3 and N-4 are localized and not engaged in resonance, making both of these options the most nucleophilic. However, the N-4 nitrogen, being a secondary nitrogen, is more sterically hindered and therefore less nucleophilic than the primary N-3 nitrogen (eliminate choice D).

5. **A** The nature of the substituents on each ring act to stabilize or destabilize the carbocation that forms. The methoxy substituent in choice A is an electron-donating group, which will stabilize the carbocation through resonance due to the lone electron pairs on the oxygen.

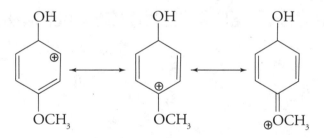

On the other hand, the nitro group in choice B will destabilize the intermediate since one resonance structure, shown below, puts two atoms with a positive charge next to each other (eliminate choice B). Choice C affords no increase or decrease in stability. Choice D will show mild stabilization due to the inductive donation offered by its methyl group (also shown below).

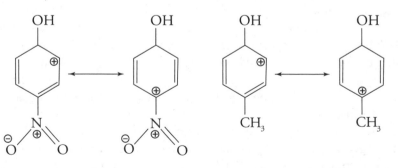

Overall, choice A shows the strongest carbocation stabilization since resonance effects are generally stronger than inductive ones.

Chapter 5
Lab Techniques:
Separations and
Spectroscopy

5.1 SEPARATIONS

Extractions

One of the more useful techniques in experimental organic chemistry is solvent extraction. Isolation of natural products from marine organisms, plants, and other natural sources is facilitated by exploiting the particular solubilities of organic compounds in various solvents. Complex mixtures of organic compounds can be separated using careful choice of solvents based on the differential solubilities of the various components of the mixture. We'll see that the acid/base properties of organic molecules play an important role in the extraction process.

Extraction allows the chemist to separate one substance from a mixture of substances by adding a solvent in which the compound of interest is highly soluble. If the solution containing the compound of interest is shaken with a second solvent (completely immiscible with the first) and allowed to separate into two distinct phases, the compound of interest will distribute itself between the two phases based upon its solubility in each of the individual solvents. This is called a **liquid-liquid extraction**. The ratio of the substance's solubilities in the two solvents is called the **distribution** (or **partition**) **coefficient**.

Solubility largely depends on two things: the polarity of the solute and the polarity of the solvent. When it comes to solubility, *like dissolves like*. Polar molecules are soluble in polar solvents, and nonpolar molecules are soluble in nonpolar solvents. For example, water is a polar solvent and hydrocarbons are nonpolar molecules. Hydrocarbons will therefore have very low solubility in water.

The simplest liquid-liquid extraction is accomplished when an organic compound is extracted with water. A simple water extraction can remove substances that are highly polar or charged, including inorganic salts, strong acids and bases, and polar, low molecular weight compounds (less than five carbons) such as alcohols, amines, and carboxylic acids.

A second class of organic extraction involves the use of acidic or basic water solutions. Organic compounds that are basic (e.g., amines) can be extracted from mixtures of organic compounds upon treatment with dilute acid (usually 5–10% HCl). This treatment will protonate the basic functional group, forming a positively charged ion. The resulting cationic salts of these basic compounds are usually freely soluble in aqueous solution and can be removed from the organic compounds that remain dissolved in the organic phase.

Extraction of Organic Amines

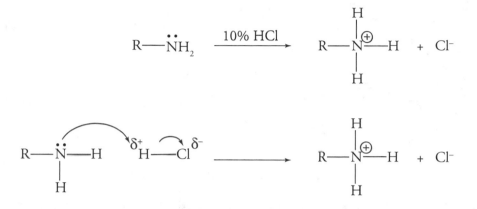

On the other hand, extraction with a dilute weak base—typically 5 percent sodium bicarbonate ($NaHCO_3$) —results in converting carboxylic acids into their corresponding anionic salts.

Extraction of Carboxylic Acids

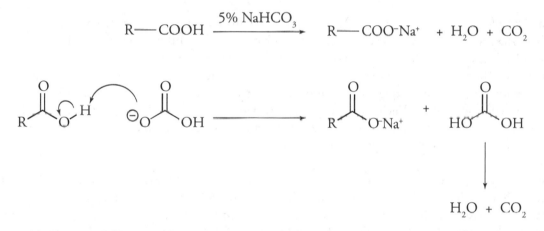

These anionic salts are generally soluble in aqueous solution and can be removed from the organic compounds that remain dissolved in the organic phase. Dilute sodium hydroxide could also be used for this kind of extraction, but it is basic enough to also convert phenols into their corresponding anionic salts. When phenols are present in a mixture of organic compounds and need to be removed, a dilute sodium hydroxide solution (usually about 10%) will succeed in converting phenols into their corresponding anionic salts. The anionic salts of the phenols are generally soluble in the aqueous phase and can therefore be removed from the organic phase.

Extraction of Phenols

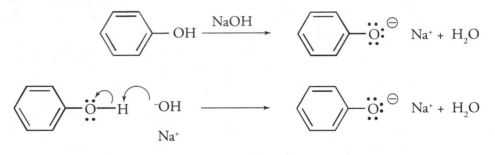

(*Note:* NaOH will also extract carboxylic acids.)

The apparatus in which these extractions are typically carried out is called a **separatory funnel**. To perform a solvent-solvent extraction, the solution containing the mixture of organic compounds and the extraction solvent of choice are poured into the separatory funnel, and the apparatus is fitted with a stopper. After mixing, the two layers may be separated from one another by removing the stopper at the top and slowly collecting each phase into separate receiving flasks by opening the stopcock at the bottom of the funnel.

As an example, let us step through an extraction that will separate four organic compounds from one another. The original mixture consists of *para*-cresol, benzoic acid, aniline, and naphthalene, all of which are dissolved in diethyl ether. This mixture is first extracted with an equal volume of aqueous sodium bicarbonate. The weakly basic bicarbonate is sufficiently basic to deprotonate benzoic acid and convert it to an anionic salt, but not strong enough to deprotonate *para*-cresol (a phenol). Likewise, a bicarbonate extraction will not affect aniline (a base itself) or naphthalene (a hydrocarbon). Thus, *para*-cresol, aniline, and naphthalene will remain dissolved in the ether phase, while the benzoic acid, now in its anionic salt form, will be extracted into the aqueous layer.

The ether layer, which now contains three components, is extracted with a sodium hydroxide solution. The strongly basic hydroxide ion is strong enough to deprotonate *para*-cresol and convert it to its anionic salt form. The basic conditions will not affect aniline or naphthalene, so *para*-cresol is the only compound that is extracted into the aqueous phase. The aniline and naphthalene will remain dissolved in the ether layer.

Finally, the remaining two components can be separated from one another by an acidic extraction with a 10% HCl solution. The solution is acidic enough to protonate the lone pair of electrons of aniline and to convert aniline to its cationic salt. Naphthalene will not be affected and will remain dissolved in the ether layer. The final extraction of aniline into the aqueous phase completes the separation. Naphthalene can be isolated by evaporating off the diethyl ether.

These steps are summarized on the following page.

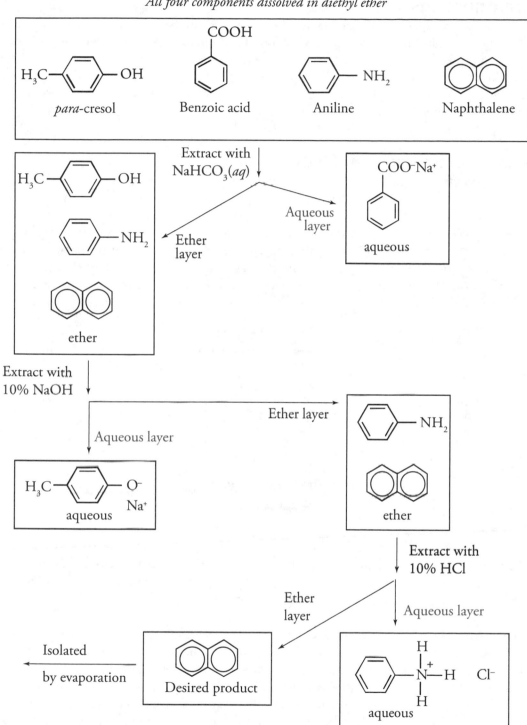

All four components dissolved in diethyl ether

para-cresol

Benzoic acid

Aniline

Naphthalene

Extract with
NaHCO$_3$(aq)

Aqueous
layer

Ether
layer

COO⁻Na⁺

aqueous

ether

Extract with
10% NaOH

Aqueous layer

Ether layer

H$_3$C——O⁻
Na⁺

aqueous

ether

Extract with
10% HCl

Ether
layer

Aqueous layer

Isolated
by evaporation

Desired product

Cl⁻

aqueous

Chromatography

While there are many types of chromatography, they all have a number of basic features in common. All types of chromatography are used to separate mixtures of compounds, though some are used mostly for identification purposes, while others are generally used as purification methods. First, we will consider thin-layer chromatography to outline the basic features. Then we will describe several other types, highlighting for each how the separation process works and the types of compounds that are most commonly separated by that method.

Thin-Layer Chromatography (TLC)

In TLC, compounds are separated based on differing polarities. Because of the speed of separation and the small sample amounts that can be successfully analyzed, this technique is frequently used in organic chemistry laboratories. Thin-layer chromatography is a solid-liquid partitioning technique in which the **mobile liquid phase** ascends a thin layer of absorbant (generally silica, SiO_2) that is coated onto a supporting material such as a glass plate. This thin layer of absorbant acts as a **polar stationary phase** for the sample to interact with. To perform TLC, a very small amount (about 1 microliter) of sample is spotted near the base of the plate (about 1 cm from the bottom) before placing the plate upright in a sealed container with a shallow layer of solvent.

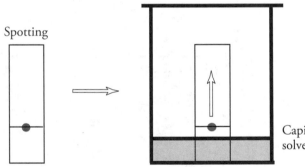

Developing the plate

Spotting

Capillary action draws the solvent up the plate.

As the solvent slowly ascends the plate via capillary action, the components of the spotted sample are partitioned between the mobile phase and the stationary phase. This process is referred to as **developing**, or **running**, a thin layer plate. Each component of the sample experiences many equilibrations between the mobile and the stationary phases as the development proceeds.

Separation of the compounds occurs because different components travel along the plate at different rates. The more polar components of the mixture interact more with the polar stationary phase and travel at a slower rate. The less polar components have a greater affinity for the solvent than the stationary phase and travel with the mobile solvent at a faster rate than the more polar components. Once the solvent nearly reaches the top of the plate, the plate is removed and allowed to dry. If the compounds in the mixture are colored, we would see a vertical series of spots on the plate; however, it is more likely that the components are not colored and need to be detected by some other means. Visualization methods include shining ultraviolet light on the plate, placing the thin layer plate in the presence of iodine vapor, and a host of other chemical staining techniques.

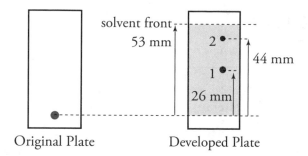

Original Plate   Developed Plate

Once the separated components have been visualized, R_f values can be computed. This "ratio to front" value (R_f) is simply the distance traveled by an individual component divided by the distance traveled by the solvent front. For example, from the illustration above, we would find

$$R_f \text{ (Compound 1)} = \frac{26 \text{ mm}}{53 \text{ mm}} = 0.49 \qquad R_f \text{ (Compound 2)} = \frac{44 \text{ mm}}{53 \text{ mm}} = 0.83$$

(Note that R_f is always positive and never greater than 1.)

Column (Flash) Chromatography

While TLC is a good technique for separating very small amounts of material in order to assess how many compounds make up a mixture, it's not a good technique for isolating bulk compounds. A common technique known as column or flash chromatography employs the same principles behind TLC toward just such a goal. Shown below is a chromatography column. This column is filled with silica gel (predominantly SiO_2, as in the TLC plate). The silica gel is saturated with a chosen organic solvent, and the mixture of compounds to be separated is then added to the top and allowed to travel down through the silica-packed column. Excess solvent is periodically added to the top of the column, and the flow of solvent (along with the separated compounds) is collected from the bottom. Just as is the case in TLC, polar compounds will spend more time adsorbed on the polar solid phase, and as such travel more slowly down the column than nonpolar compounds. Therefore, compounds can be expected to leave the column, and be collected, in order of polarity (least polar to most polar).

Column Chromatography

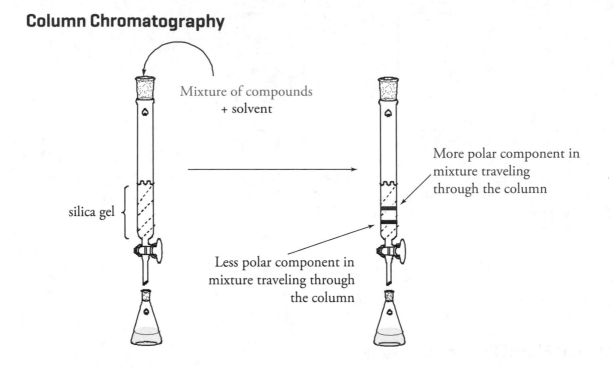

Ion Exchange Chromatography

In applications where the materials to be separated have varying charge states, ion exchange chromatography may be employed. This method, again involving passing a mobile liquid phase containing the analyte through a column packed with a solid stationary phase, utilizes a polymeric resin functionalized with either positive or negatively charged moieties on the polymer surface.

The schematic below depicts the passage of an analyte containing both positively and negatively charged ionic species, as well neutral molecules, through a pore of an ion exchange resin. The particular stationary phase resin depicted below is functionalized with anionic sulfonate groups, initially coordinated to sodium cations.

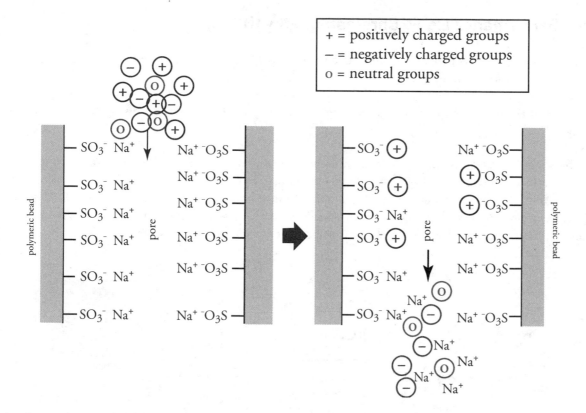

As the analyte passes through the resin, positively charged groups displace sodium ions and coordinate to the anionic functionalities tethered to the polymer surface. While these groups are retained, and their progress through the column retarded, the negatively charged groups and neutral species quickly pass through the material and are eluted first. Once all the negatively charged and neutral species have been eluted, the column can be treated with a concentrated sodium-containing solution to displace all adsorbed positively charged species.

Ion exchange chromatography is frequently used in the separation of mixtures of proteins. At any given pH, proteins within a mixture may exist in a variety of charge states (more on this in Chapter 7). If such a mixture is passed through a cation exchange resin (one functionalized with negatively charged groups and cationic counterions as shown in the figure above), those proteins with pI values greater than the pH of the mobile phase will be positively charged and elute slowly compared to those with pI values below the solution pH. If the same mixture at the same pH were passed through an anion exchange resin, the opposite would be true, and proteins with pI values above the pH of the solution will elute first. If the pI values of the proteins to be separated are known, the pH of the mobile phase may be buffered to a specific pH, thereby ensuring different charge states and hence good separation.

High Performance Liquid Chromatography (HPLC)

HPLC uses the same principles as all chromatographic separation techniques, and takes advantage of the differing affinities of various compounds for either a stationary phase or a mobile phase. However, because the mobile phase is forced through the stationary phase at very high pressures, both the speed and efficiency of the separation is increased, making this technique an improvement over column chromatography.

The basic configuration of an HPLC system is shown in the figure below. The pumping unit is where pressurization of the mobile phase first occurs. The sample to be separated is solubilized and injected by syringe, then the mobile phase carries the sample to the column. The sample is separated into its constituent components, which are detected and analyzed as they exit the column. The eluent is collected after detection, and the components can be isolated after evaporation of the solvent, if desired.

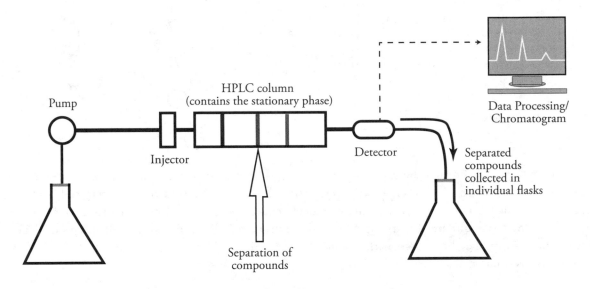

The elution time of any compound is dependent upon the mobile and stationary phases used. For most HPLC separations of organic compounds, the stationary phase is a silica gel that has been bonded to a nonpolar group (e.g., octadecylsilane), creating a relatively *nonpolar* stationary phase. This is called reverse phase HPLC. The mobile phase used is generally *more polar* than the stationary phase. This means the order of elution will be the reverse of what occurs on a TLC plate or in simple column chromatography. More polar compounds elute first in HPLC as they have a high affinity for the mobile phase. The less polar compounds are slowed by their interactions with the nonpolar stationary phase, and therefore elute last.

For the analysis of charged compounds, such as amino acids, the stationary phase is often an ion exchange column, usually cation exchange. The mobile phase is a polar, protic (e.g, CH_3OH or H_2O) or acidic solvent that ensures solubility and suppresses the dissociation of the COOH group on the amino acid. The difference in affinity to the column is attributed to the effects of the various R groups of the amino acids. Elution order can be predicted based on an analysis of the intermolecular forces of these side chains.

Size Exclusion Chromatography

Size exclusion chromatography is a technique used to separate bulk materials based on molecular size. Much like flash chromatography, the materials to be separated are dissolved in solvent, loaded onto a column packed with a stationary phase, and allowed to travel to the bottom of the column where they are collected.

In contrast to flash chromatography, which uses a polar silicate stationary phase, the stationary phase employed in size exclusion chromatography most often consists of chemically inert, porous polymer beads. The sizes of the pores in the bead are carefully controlled to allow permeation of small molecules in the eluent, while excluding larger ones. A schematic for the beads and the paths taken by large and small molecules is depicted below.

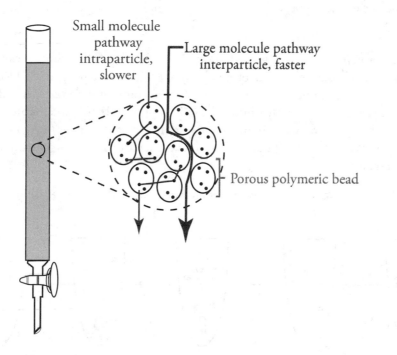

The exclusion of large molecules from the pore volume creates a more direct path down the column for large species than the more complicated intraparticle pathway taken by compounds small enough to permeate the beads. The overall result is the quick elution of large molecules and longer retention of smaller species.

Size exclusion chromatography is frequently used for the separation of large polymers from small oligiomeric fragments, or the separation of full proteins from smaller peptide chains. The lack of chemical interaction between the mobile and stationary phases results in relatively speedy elution (compared to chromatography on silica) and minimal loss of material on the column. However, though materials of very different sizes are easily separated, the technique is not particularly effective at separating different compounds of similar sizes.

Affinity Chromatography

Affinity chromatography is most commonly used to purify proteins or nucleic acids from complex biochemical mixtures like cell lysates, growth media, or blood, rather than a reaction mixture. It is based on highly specific interactions between macromolecules. As a result of this specific binding, the target molecule is trapped on the stationary phase, which is then washed to remove the unwanted components of the mixture. The target protein is then released (or eluted) off the solid phase in a highly purified state.

In large-scale work, the stationary phase is a column packed with a solid resin, and the sample is poured through the column. In smaller scale experiments, the solid phase can be mixed in a small tube with the sample to allow interaction with the components of the mixture. The sample is then centrifuged (spun at high speeds) so the heavy solid resin settles to the bottom of the tube. Since the protein of interest is bound to the solid resin, the liquid (or supernatant) is simply decanted, leaving the desired compound behind.

In order to isolate a protein of interest, the highly specific interactions of antibodies can be used, as shown in the figure below. A commercially available antibody specific for the protein is added to the lysate sample. To isolate the antigen-antibody complex, one of three common microbe-derived proteins (Protein A, Protein G, or Protein L) is covalently linked to a solid support. These proteins are useful because they bind mammalian antibodies, so upon mixing, complexes made of *Protein of Interest – Antibody – Protein A/G/L – Solid Support Bead* form in solution. The target is then isolated after centrifuging the sample and decanting the supernatant.

Purifying a Protein of Interest using an Antibody and Protein A-linked Beads

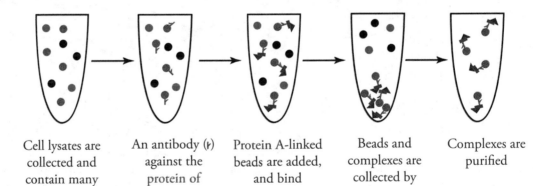

| Cell lysates are collected and contain many proteins | An antibody (⊢) against the protein of interest is added | Protein A-linked beads are added, and bind antibodies | Beads and complexes are collected by centrifugation | Complexes are purified |

Instead of centrifugation, magnetic beads can be used as the solid phase, as shown below. The beads are isolated from solution by using a magnet to hold them (bound to the protein of interest) against the sides of the tube, while the solution containing any undesired compounds is decanted. Then the desired compound can be released from the beads in a pure state.

Using Magnetic Beads as the Solid Phase in Affinity Chromatography

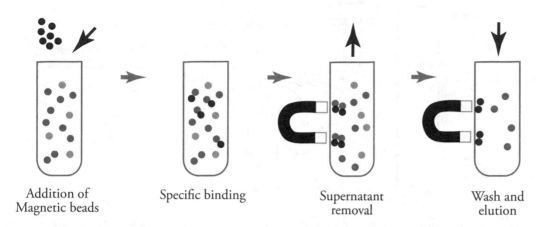

| Addition of Magnetic beads | Specific binding | Supernatant removal | Wash and elution |

Not all proteins of interest have a commercial antibody available. In this case, researchers can use an **affinity tag**. Using recombinant technology (described in Appendix 1 of the MCAT Biology Review), a small molecular tag is added to the N-terminus or the C-terminus of the protein. DNA sequences coding for affinity tags are well known, and these can be subcloned into a plasmid with the gene of interest. Affinity-tagged proteins can be produced in large amounts in laboratory bacteria, and the cell lysate collected is rich in tagged protein.

There are many types of affinity tags, and they are generally small enough that they don't interfere with protein folding or function. One class of commonly used affinity tags are the His tags (made of 6-10 histidine amino acids), which bind ions such as nickel. When a cell lysate is applied to a column packed with nickel-based resin, the His-tagged proteins bind to the resin. This is done under high pH conditions, and the His-tagged protein can be eluted off the solid phase using lower pH conditions.

Gas Chromatography

Gas chromatography (GC) is a form of column chromatography in which the partitioning of the components to be separated takes place between a **mobile gas phase** and a **stationary liquid phase**. This partitioning, or separation, between mixtures of compounds occurs based on their *different volatilities*. In a typical gas chromatograph, a sample is loaded into a syringe and injected into the device through a rubber septum. The sample is then vaporized by a heater in the injection port and carried along by a stream of inert gas (typically helium). The vaporized sample is quickly moved by the inert gas stream into a column composed of particles that are coated with a liquid absorbant. As the components of the sample pass through the column, they interact differently with the absorbant based on their relative volatilities. Each component of the sample is subjected to many gas-liquid partitioning processes which separates the individual components.

As each component exits the column, it is burned, and the resulting ions are detected by an electrical detector that generates a signal that is recorded by a chart recorder. The chart recorder printout enables us to determine the number of components and their relative amounts.

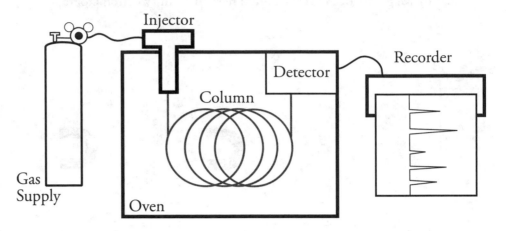

Let's now take a closer look at the separation process by examining a typical GC column. To do so, we will consider a mixture of two individual components. As the mixture enters the column, it begins to interact with the stationary phase, which is composed of support material coated with a liquid absorbant. The liquid absorbants can range from hydrocarbon mixtures that are very nonpolar to polyesters that are polar. As the mixture passes through the column, the components equilibrate between the carrier gas and the liquid phase. The less volatile components will spend more time dissolved in the liquid stationary phase than the more volatile component that will be carried along by the carrier gas at a faster rate. It is this equilibrium between the component (the absorbed liquid phase and the carrier gas mobile phase) that results in the separation of the mixture. If the interactions of the substrates with the column are similar (this is usually the case with most GC columns), the more volatile components emerge from the column first, while the less volatile components emerge from the column later.

Physical Properties of Organic Compounds

As we just discussed, it's the volatility, or boiling point, of a compound that is most important to consider when conducting a gas chromatography experiment. Generally speaking, this technique separates only small amounts of material, whereas the next technique, distillation, does the same thing, just for larger amounts of material.

In order to best understand the principles behind distillations, as well as predict when it's appropriate to use, we should first discuss some fundamentals about the physical properties of compounds, namely melting points and boiling points, and how they are related to the intermolecular forces of molecules.

Melting and Boiling Points

Melting point (mp) and **boiling point (bp)** are indicators of how well identical molecules interact with (attract) each other. Nonpolar molecules, like hydrocarbons, interact principally because of an attractive force known as the London dispersion force, one of the intermolecular (van der Waals) forces. This force exists between temporary dipoles formed in nonpolar molecules as a result of a temporary asymmetric electron distribution. Such intermolecular forces must be overcome to melt a nonpolar compound (solid → liquid) or to boil a nonpolar compound (liquid → gas). The greater the attractive forces between molecules, the more energy will be required to get the compound to melt or boil. The weaker these forces, the lower the melting or boiling point.

Many factors determine the degree to which molecules of a given compound will interact. For hydrocarbons, the most significant of these factors is *branching*. Branching tends to inhibit van der Waals forces by reducing the surface area available for intermolecular interaction. Thus, branching tends to reduce attractive forces between molecules and to lower both melting point and boiling point. Consider the following two constitutional isomers:

Molecule I
n-octane

Molecule II
2,4-dimethylhexane

Molecule I, *n*-octane, is unbranched. Molecule II, 2,4-dimethylhexane, is a branched isomer of *n*-octane. Although each compound has the same molecular formula, C_8H_{18}, these two constitutional isomers have dramatically different melting points and boiling points. *n*-Octane requires much more energy to melt or boil, because unbranched, it experiences greater van der Waals forces than does the branched isomer 2,4-dimethylhexane. Therefore, *n*-octane has both a higher melting point and a higher boiling point than does 2,4-dimethylhexane.

The second factor influencing melting point and boiling point for hydrocarbons is molecular weight. The greater the molecular weight of a compound, the more surface area there is to interact, the greater the number of van der Waals interactions, and the higher the melting point and boiling point. Therefore, hexane—a six-carbon alkane—has a higher mp and bp than propane, a three-carbon alkane.

The influence of molecular weight on melting point and boiling point is readily seen when considering the following trends for hydrocarbons:

- Small hydrocarbons (1 to 4 carbons) tend to be gases at room temperature.
- Intermediate hydrocarbons (5 to 16 carbons) tend to be liquids at room temperature.
- Large hydrocarbons (more than 16 carbons) tend to be (waxy) solids at room temperature.

Example 5-1: Rank the following six hydrocarbons in order of increasing boiling point:

Solution: Since branching lowers the boiling point, each of the branched hydrocarbons has a lower boiling point than the unbranched hydrocarbon of the same molecular formula. Also, the larger the molecule, the greater the surface area over which van der Waals forces can act, so heavier molecules have higher boiling points. We can now put the whole sequence in order of increasing bp:

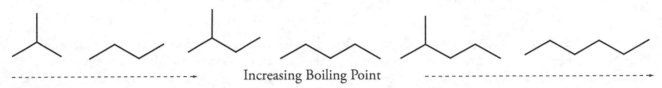

Increasing Boiling Point

Hydrogen Bonding

Another important type of intermolecular force that has a large effect on the physical properties of organic molecules is the hydrogen bond. In order to examine the effect of hydrogen bonding on melting or boiling points, let's examine two molecules that are isomers of one another, *n*-butanol and diethyl ether. Both have the same molecular formula ($C_4H_{10}O$), yet there is a dramatic difference in their boiling points (117°C for *n*-butanol vs. 34.6°C for diethyl ether). This difference arises from the ability of *n*-butanol to form intermolecular hydrogen bonds, while diethyl ether *cannot*.

Recall from General Chemistry that hydrogen bonding occurs between a hydrogen-bond donor—a hydrogen covalently bonded to a nitrogen, oxygen, or fluorine atom, and a hydrogen-bond acceptor—a lone pair of electrons on a nitrogen, oxygen, or fluorine in another molecule, or part of the first molecule. Alcohols form intermolecular hydrogen bonds because they have hydroxyl (–OH) groups. This results from a strong dipole in which the hydroxyl group's hydrogen acquires a substantial partial positive charge (δ^+) and the oxygen acquires a substantial partial negative charge (δ^-). The partial positive hydrogen can interact electrostatically with a non-bonding pair of electrons on a nearby oxygen, resulting in a hydrogen bond.

On the other hand, diethyl ether has an oxygen atom with non-bonding electrons but all hydrogen atoms are bound to carbons. Since carbon and hydrogen have similar electronegativity values, the bond is not very polarized, and these hydrogens cannot participate in hydrogen bonding. It's important to remember that a hydrogen bond is *not* a covalent bond; in this case it's an intermolecular interaction.

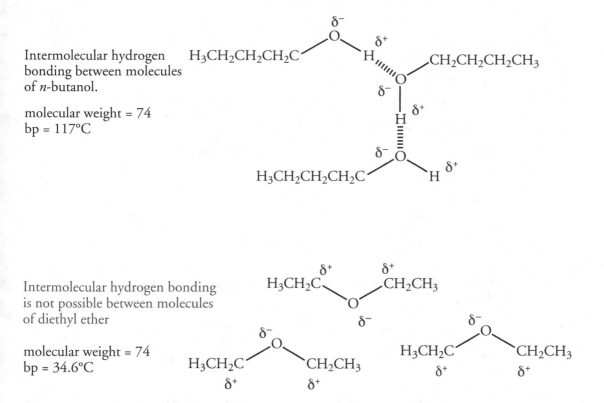

Intermolecular hydrogen bonding between molecules of *n*-butanol.

molecular weight = 74
bp = 117°C

Intermolecular hydrogen bonding is not possible between molecules of diethyl ether

molecular weight = 74
bp = 34.6°C

The hydrogen bonding pattern in phenols provides insight into *inter*molecular vs. *intra*molecular hydrogen bonding. Let's consider the two isomers, 4-nitrophenol and 2-nitrophenol. First, examine the hydrogen bonding pattern in 4-nitrophenol. Notice that hydrogen bonding can occur with both the nitro and the hydroxyl groups in this molecule and that the bonding is exclusively intermolecular. That is, all hydrogen bonding takes place between individual molecules of 4-nitrophenol. These hydrogen bonding interactions hold molecules of 4-nitrophenol together and increase their boiling and melting points.

Now, examine the hydrogen bonding pattern in 2-nitrophenol. Notice that for this molecule, the nitro group and the hydroxyl group are in close proximity so that intramolecular hydrogen bonding can occur between the hydrogen of the hydroxyl group and a lone pair of electrons on the nitro group *on the same molecule*. These intramolecular hydrogen bonding interactions decrease the amount of intermolecular hydrogen bonding interactions that can occur between molecules thereby decreasing the melting and boiling points of 2-nitrophenol (46°C) relative to 4-nitrophenol (114°C).

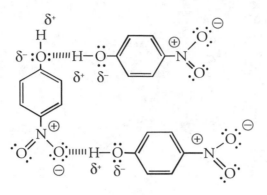

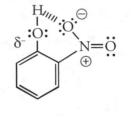

4-nitrophenol
Intermolecular hydrogen bonding

2-nitrophenol
Intramolecular hydrogen bonding

Example 5-2: Rank the following three compounds in order of increasing boiling point:

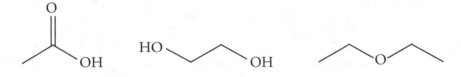

Solution: The more hydrogen-bond donors and hydrogen-bond acceptors there are in a molecule, the higher the boiling and melting points will be. This is because the hydrogen bonds, like dispersion forces, act to *hold* the molecules together, resisting the change to becoming either a liquid or a gas. The first molecule, acetic acid ($C_2H_4O_2$), has one hydrogen-bond donor and four hydrogen-bond acceptors. The second molecule, 1,2-ethanediol ($C_2H_6O_2$), has two hydrogen-bond donors and four hydrogen-bond acceptors. The third molecule, diethyl ether ($C_4H_{10}O$), has two hydrogen-bond acceptors, but no hydrogen bond donors. From this we can now correctly assign the order of their boiling points:

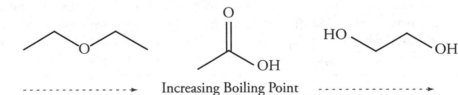

- - - - - - - - - - - -▸   Increasing Boiling Point   - - - - - - - - - - - -▸

Example 5-3: For each of the following pairs of compounds, predict which molecule will have the higher boiling point.

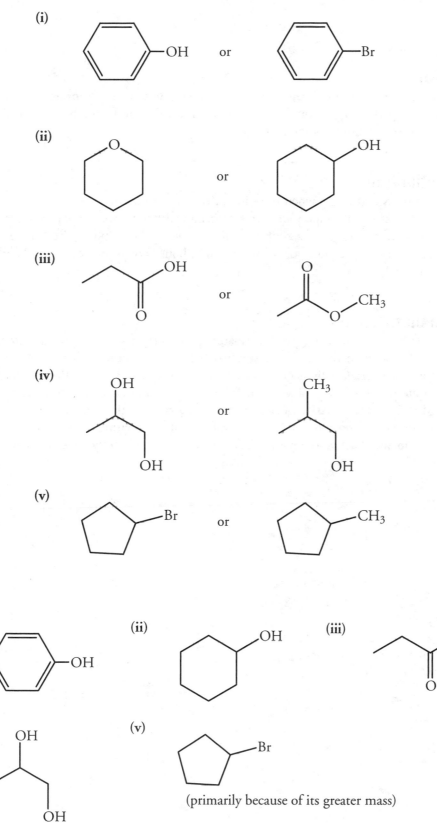

(i)

(ii)

(iii)

(iv)

(v)

Solution:

(i)

(ii)

(iii)

(iv)

(v)

(primarily because of its greater mass)

With a better understanding of what helps to determine the boiling point of an organic molecule, let's now discuss the next important separation technique for the MCAT—distillations.

Distillations

Distillation is the process of raising the temperature of a liquid until it can overcome the intermolecular forces that hold it together in the liquid phase. The vapor is then condensed back to the liquid phase and subsequently collected in another container.

Simple Distillation

A simple distillation is performed when trace impurities need to be removed from a relatively pure compound, or when a mixture of compounds with significantly different boiling points needs to be separated. For example, an appropriate use of a simple distillation would be to purify fresh drinking water away from a salt water solution. The more volatile water can be boiled away, then condensed and collected, leaving behind the nonvolatile salts.

Fractional Distillation

Fractional distillation is a different type of distillation process that is used when the difference in boiling points of the components in the liquid mixture is not large. A fractional distillation column is packed with an appropriate material, such as glass beads or a stainless steel sponge. The packing of the column results in the liquid mixture being subjected to many vaporization-condensation cycles as it moves up the column toward the condenser. As the cycles progress, the composition of the vapor gradually becomes enriched in the lower boiling component. Near the top of the column, nearly pure vapor reaches the condenser and condenses back to the liquid phase where it is subsequently collected in a receiving flask.

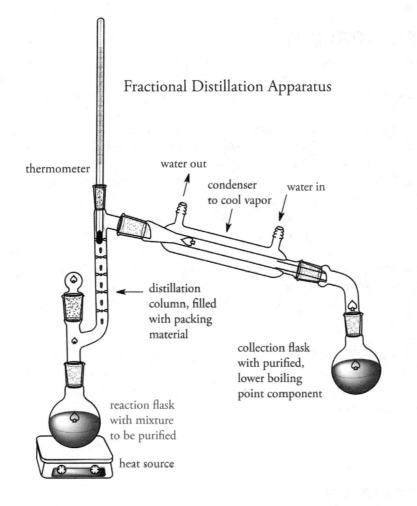

Fractional Distillation Apparatus

thermometer

water out

condenser
to cool vapor

water in

distillation
column, filled
with packing
material

collection flask
with purified,
lower boiling
point component

reaction flask
with mixture
to be purified

heat source

Example 5-4: A chemist wishes to separate a mixture of Compounds A and B. He decides to distill the mixture; however, he is unsure of their respective boiling points. After several minutes of heating, he collects the distillate, takes a small sample, and injects it into a gas chromatograph. The output is:

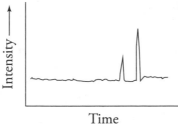

What can this chemist conclude about the separation, and how could it be improved?

Solution: Based on the data from the GC, his separation was only partial (because two different peaks are recorded). Because the second peak is larger than the first, the distillate consists primarily of one of the two compounds, but their boiling points may have been similar enough such that a complete separation was not possible. Perhaps the chemist should try fractional distillation.

5.2 SPECTROSCOPY

A basic understanding of the general principles of spectroscopy will enable you to answer important questions regarding the structure of organic molecules. In this section, we'll examine the general principles of spectroscopy with the goal of interpreting the spectra of simple organic molecules.

Most types of spectroscopy that we will discuss are examples of absorption spectroscopy. A short explanation of the molecular events involved in absorption spectroscopy will help you remember the details of IR and NMR spectroscopy. Molecules normally exist in their lowest energy form, called their **ground state**. When a molecule is exposed to light it *may* absorb a photon, provided the energy of this photon matches the energy between two of the fixed electronic energy levels of the molecule. When this happens, the molecule is said to be in an **excited state**. Molecules tend to prefer their ground state to an excited state, but in order for them to return to their ground state, they must lose the energy they have gained. This loss of energy can occur by the emission of heat, or less commonly, light. In absorption spectroscopy, scientists induce the absorption of energy by a sample of molecules by exposing the sample to various forms of light, thereby exciting molecules to a higher energy state. They then measure the energy released as the molecules relax back to their ground state. This measured energy can reveal structural features of the molecules in the sample.

There are many different forms of light, as displayed in the electromagnetic spectrum. In principle, any of these forms of light could be used to do absorption spectroscopy on molecules, and, in fact, many are! The different forms of light induce different transitions in ground state molecules to different excited states of the molecules and allow for the acquisition of different structural information about the molecules.

Mass Spectrometry

Mass spectrometry is a very useful technique that allows researchers to determine the mass of compounds in a sample. Within the mass spectrometer, molecules are ionized in a high vacuum, usually by bombarding them with high energy electrons. Once ionized, compounds enter a region of the spectrometer where they are acted on by a magnetic field. This field causes the flight path of the charged species to alter, and the degree to which the path is changed is determined by the mass of the ion. This difference is detected and translated into a mass readout in the detector.

On the following page is a schematic of a portion of the mass spectrum for *n*-nonane (MW = 128 g/mol).

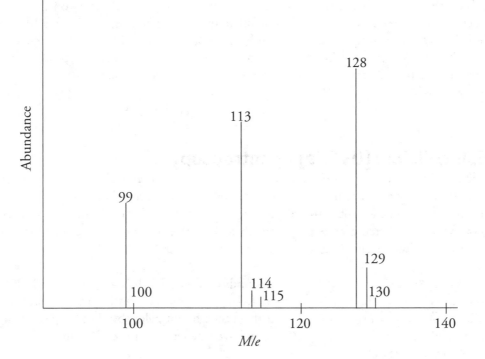

The M/e label on the x-axis represents the ratio of mass (M) to charge (e). In most cases e = +1, so peaks can simply be viewed as molecular mass. The y-axis represents the relative abundance of each species of a particular mass detected in the sample. Masses, though generally not labeled as such, are measured in amu.

Two aspects of the above spectrum may be puzzling: 1) If the molecular weight of nonane is 128 g/mol, why are there peaks greater than this value, and 2) why are there significant peaks in the sample with masses lower than 128?

Remember, atoms can come in a number of different isotopes. For example, the most prevalent mass of hydrogen in nature is 1, but deuterium has an extra neutron and weighs 2 (natural abundance = .015%). Likewise, the most abundant isotope of carbon is ^{12}C, but ^{13}C exists as 1.1% of all carbon atoms. So, the small peaks with masses larger than the main peak represent molecules that have one or more of these less abundant isotopes.

The masses lower than 128 in the above scan represent the masses of molecular fragments. The high-energy beam of electrons used to ionize molecules in the mass spectrometer can cause the molecule to break into smaller parts. The figure below shows where n-nonane might have been broken to produce peaks with the masses found above. The outer, curved brackets represent a fragment which has lost the terminal CH_3 group and hence is 15 less than the peak at 128. The inner, square brackets show a fragment weighing 99, having lost CH_2CH_3.

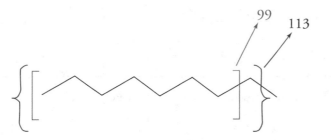

5.2

Particular atoms present in a molecule may give characteristic peaks in their mass spectra thanks to isotopic ratios. The two most important are Br and Cl. Bromine naturally occurs in two isotopes (79 and 81) of nearly identical natural abundance. This means that any mass spectrum involving a brominated compound will have two major peaks, nearly equal in height, 2 amu apart. Chlorine also occurs as two main isotopes; 35 (75% natural abundance) and 37 (25% natural abundance). Mass spectra for chlorinated molecules will have a peak 2 amu heavier than the main peak, and about one-third its height.

Ultraviolet/Visible (UV/Vis) Spectroscopy

UV/Vis spectroscopy is a type of absorption spectroscopy used in organic chemistry. It is very similar to IR (which we'll discuss next), but instead focuses on the slightly shorter, more energetic wavelengths of radiation in the ultraviolet and visible area of the spectrum. The wavelengths in the UV and visible ranges of the electromagnetic spectrum are strong enough to induce electronic excitation, promoting ground state valence electrons into excited states.

In general, UV/Vis spectroscopy is used with two kinds of molecules. It is very useful in monitoring complexes of transition metals. The easy promotion of electrons from ground to excited states in the closely spaced d-orbitals of many transition metals gives them their bright color (by absorbing wavelengths in the visible region), and since many of these promotions involve energies in the UV range, these promotions allow study of these species.

More importantly in organic chemistry, UV/Vis spectroscopy is used to study highly conjugated organic systems. Molecular orbital theory tells us that when molecules have conjugated π-systems, orbitals form many bonding, non-bonding, and anti-bonding orbitals. These orbitals can be reasonably close together in energy, and in fact, close enough to allow promotion of electrons between electronic states through absorption of ultraviolet, or even visible photons. The wavelength of maximum absorption for any compound is directly related to the extent of conjugation in the molecule. The more extensive the conjugated system is, the longer the wavelength of maximum absorption will be. To illustrate this relationship, let's look at a series of polycyclic aromatic hydrocarbons in Table 5.1 below.

		λ_{max}	absorbs	appears
Anthracene		363 nm	UV	white
Tetracene		475 nm	blue	orange
Pentacene		595 nm	yellow/orange	blue/violet

Table 5.1 UV/Vis Spectroscopic Data for Select Polycyclic Aromatic Hydrocarbons

With the addition of each aromatic ring, the conjugated system grows longer and the wavelength of maximum absorption increases. Since each λ_{max} corresponds to a particular color of light, a simple color wheel can be used to predict the color the compound will appear. As a general rule, the color a compound maximally absorbs is complementary to the color it will appear to our eyes. For a compound that absorbs only ultraviolet radiation, ALL of the visible wavelengths will be reflected and thus the compound will appear white or colorless. However, a compound that absorbs blue light will appear to us as orange, since blue and orange are complementary colors on opposites sides of the color wheel (Figure 5.1).

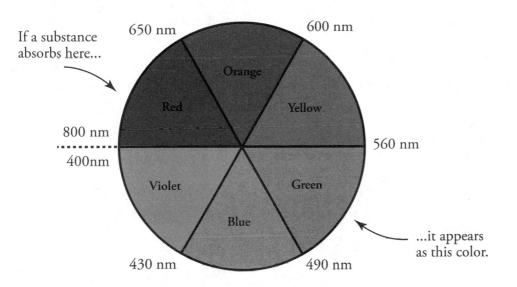

Figure 5.1 Color Wheel Showing Complementary Colors

Infrared (IR) Spectroscopy

Electromagnetic radiation in the infrared (IR) range λ = 2.5 to 20 μm has the proper energy to cause bonds in organic molecules to become vibrationally excited. When a sample of an organic compound is irradiated with infrared radiation in the region between 2.5 and 20 μm, its covalent bonds will begin to *vibrate at distinct energy levels* (wavelengths, frequencies) within this region. These wavelengths correspond to frequencies in the range of 1.5×10^{13} Hz to 1.2×10^{14} Hz. In IR spectroscopy, vibrational frequencies are more commonly given in terms of the **wavenumber**. Wavenumber ($\overline{v}$) is simply the reciprocal of wavelength:

$$\overline{v} = \frac{1}{\lambda} = \frac{1}{c}v$$

and is therefore directly proportional to both the frequency (since $\lambda v = c = 3 \times 10^{10}$ cm/sec) and the energy of the radiation (since $E = hv$). That is, the higher the wavenumber, the higher the frequency and the greater the energy. Wavenumbers are usually expressed in *reciprocal centimeters*, cm⁻¹, and MCAT IR spectra will typically cover the range from 4000 to 1000 cm⁻¹.

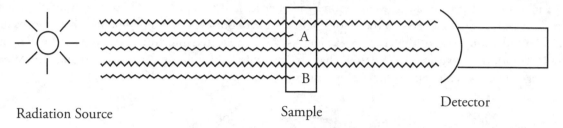

Radiation Source   Sample   Detector

When a bond absorbs IR radiation of a specific frequency, that frequency is not recorded by the detector and is thus seen as a peak in the IR spectrum (since low transmittance corresponds, naturally, to absorbance):

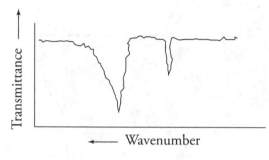

Important Stretching Frequencies

In order to do well on the MCAT, it is important that you know the stretching frequencies of the common functional groups. The most important ones are listed below.

The Double Bond Stretches

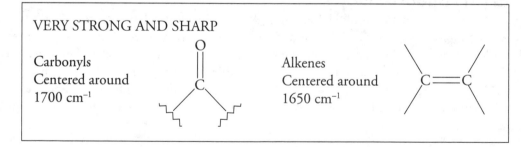

VERY STRONG AND SHARP

Carbonyls
Centered around
1700 cm⁻¹

Alkenes
Centered around
1650 cm⁻¹

We'll begin by examining the carbonyl, or C=O, stretch. The carbonyl stretch is centered around 1700 cm⁻¹ and is very **strong** and very **intense**. *Strength* is reflected in the percent absorbance (or transmittance). *Intensity* is reflected in the sharpness or distinctiveness ("V" shape) of the spike appearing on the spectrum. The carbonyl stretch is one of the most important absorptions, and you should commit its location to memory. In any spectrum, always look for this stretch first. If it is *not* present, you can eliminate a wide range of compounds that contain a carbonyl group, including aldehydes, ketones, carboxylic acids, acid chlorides, esters, amides, and anhydrides. On the other hand, if the carbonyl stretch *is* present, you know that one of the carbonyl-containing functional groups is indeed present.

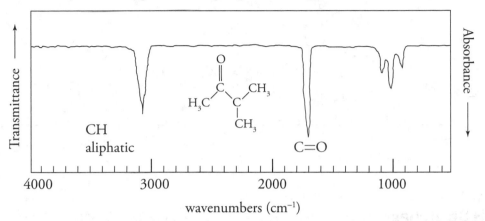

The C=C double bond stretch will appear slightly lower in the spectrum, near 1650 cm^{-1}.

The Triple Bond Stretch

The next stretch to consider is the triple bond. This is an easy one because few molecules possess these functional groups. If they are present, however, the following characteristic stretches will be seen:

$$C \equiv C \quad \text{or} \quad C \equiv N$$

2260–2100 cm^{-1}

The O—H Stretch

Next we come to the hydroxyl stretch. *The O—H stretch is strong and very broad.* **Strength** is reflected as the degree of absorption a peak displays in the spectrum. **Broadness** is reflected as a wide "U"-shaped appearance on the absorption spectrum, as opposed to a "V," or spiked shape. The broadness is due to hydrogen bonding. Like the carbonyl stretch that occurs at 1700 cm^{-1}, one should always look for the O—H stretch at 3600–3200 cm^{-1}. Amines also have stretches in this region although they vary in intensity.

O—H

3600–3200 cm^{-1}

Alcohols

5.2

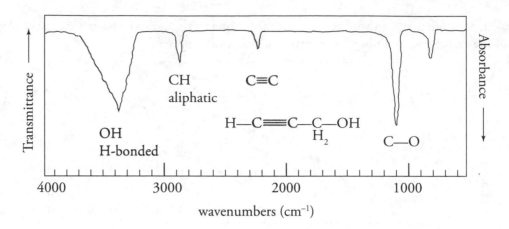

The C—H Stretches

Finally we come to the C—H stretching region (3300–2850 cm^{-1}). Since the vast majority of organic compounds contain C—H bonds, you will almost always see absorbances in this region. Note that aliphatic C—H bonds stretch at wavenumbers a little less than 3000 cm^{-1}, and aromatic C—H bonds stretch at wavenumbers slightly greater than 3000 cm^{-1}.

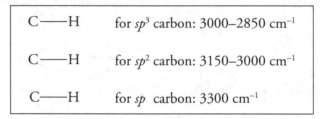

C——H	for sp^3 carbon: 3000–2850 cm^{-1}
C——H	for sp^2 carbon: 3150–3000 cm^{-1}
C——H	for sp carbon: 3300 cm^{-1}

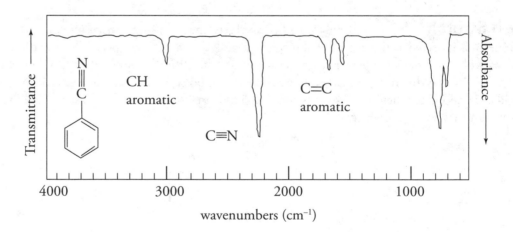

Summary of Relevant Infrared (IR) Stretching Frequencies

Bond	Frequency (Wavenumber) Range [cm^{-1}]	Intensity
C=O	1735–1680	strong
C=C	1680–1620	variable
C≡C	2260–2100	variable
C≡N	2260–2220	variable
C—H	3300–2700	variable
N—H	3150–2500	moderate
O—H	3650–3200	broad

^{1}H Nuclear Magnetic Resonance (NMR) Spectroscopy

^{1}H NMR spectroscopy, commonly called proton NMR, is the third type of absorption spectroscopy that we will consider. In all types of NMR spectroscopy, light from the radio frequency range of the electromagnetic spectrum is used to induce energy absorptions. The interpretation of ^{1}H NMR spectral data is important for the MCAT, but the theory underlying NMR spectroscopy is beyond the scope of the exam. Here, we'll only cover the interpretation of ^{1}H NMR spectra.

Four essential features of a molecule can be deduced from its ^{1}H NMR spectrum, and while we'll review all four, it is most important for the MCAT to focus on the first two. First, the number of sets of peaks in the spectrum tells one the number of chemically nonequivalent sets of protons in the molecule. Second, the splitting pattern of each set of peaks tells how many protons are interacting with the protons in that set. Third, the mathematical integration of the sets of peaks indicates the relative numbers of protons in each set. Fourth, the chemical shift values of those sets of peaks gives information about the environment of the protons in that set. These four key features of ^{1}H NMR spectroscopy are explained in the next four sections.

Chemically Equivalent Hydrogens

Determining which hydrogens, or protons, are **equivalent** in an organic molecule is the first important skill to master with respect to NMR spectroscopy. Equivalent hydrogens in a molecule are those that have *identical electronic environments*. Such hydrogens have identical locations in the ^{1}H NMR spectrum, and are therefore represented by the same signal, or resonance. Nonequivalent hydrogens will have different locations in the ^{1}H NMR spectrum and be represented by different signals. One must be able to determine which hydrogens (or, usually, groups of hydrogens) are equivalent to which other groups, so that you can predict how many distinct NMR signals there will be in any ^{1}H NMR spectrum. Hydrogens are considered equivalent if they can be interchanged by a free rotation or a symmetry operation (mirror plane or rotational axis). Check yourself on the following examples:

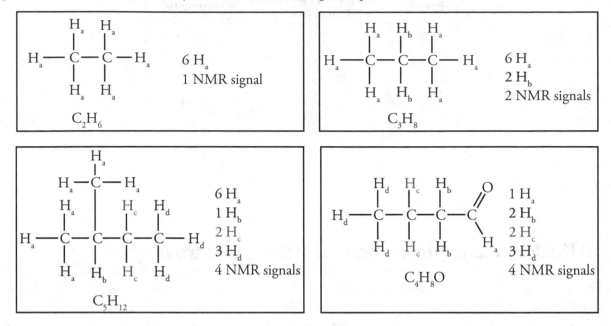

Example 5-5: A hydrocarbon C_5H_{12} shows only one peak on its ^1H NMR spectrum. Identify its structure.

Solution: Compute the degrees of unsaturation: $d = [2(\#C) + 2 - (\#H)]/2$. In this case, $d = 0$, so there are no double bonds or rings. Because there is only one peak in the ^1H NMR spectrum, all protons are equivalent, and thus our molecule must be:

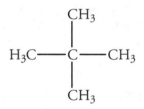

Example 5-6: C_5H_{10} also has an ^1H NMR spectrum showing only one peak. Identify its structure.

Solution: Here, $d = [2(\#C) + 2 - (\#H)]/2 = 1$, so the molecule has a double bond or ring. All C_5H_{10} variations with a double bond have more than one type of proton. But in cyclopentane, all hydrogens are equivalent due to the presence of a five-fold axis of symmetry:

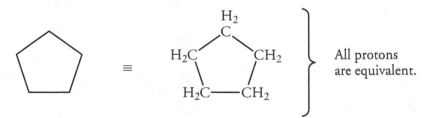

Splitting

The second aspect of NMR spectroscopy that you should be familiar with is the **spin-spin splitting phenomenon**. This occurs when nonequivalent hydrogens interact with each other. This interaction exists because the magnetic field felt by a proton is influenced by surrounding protons. This effect tends to fall off with distance, but it can often extend over two adjacent carbons. Nearby protons that are nonequivalent to the proton in question will cause a splitting in the observed ^1H NMR signal. The degree of splitting depends on the number of adjacent hydrogens, and a signal will be split into $n + 1$ lines, where n is the number of nonequivalent, neighboring (interacting) protons. The important information one must determine is how a proton or a group of chemically equivalent protons will be split by their hydrogen neighbors.

This is best demonstrated by an example:

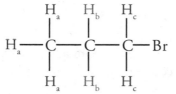

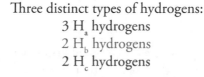

Three distinct types of hydrogens:
   3 H_a hydrogens
   2 H_b hydrogens
   2 H_c hydrogens

H_a signal split into **three** peaks due to the two neighboring, but different, H_b atoms.

H_b signal split into **six** peaks due to the five neighboring, but different, H_a and H_c atoms.

H_c signal split into **three** peaks due to the two neighboring, but different, H_b atoms.

Note that, for MCAT purposes, the H_a and H_c protons neighboring H_b do not have to be equivalent in order to add them together to get $n = 5$.

$n + 1$ RULE

n = Number of neighboring nonequivalent hydrogens	Splitting ($n + 1$)
0	1—Singlet
1	2—Doublet
2	3—Triplet
3	4—Quartet
4	5—Quintet (or multiplet)
5	6—Sextet (or multiplet)

Consider the NMR spectrum of CH_3CH_2I:

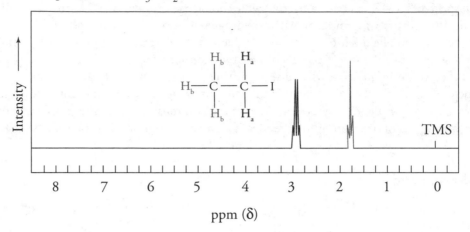

The α-hydrogens have three neighboring hydrogens and are therefore split into a quartet, according to the $n + 1$ rule. The β-hydrogens are split into a triplet because they have two neighboring hydrogens.

Example 5-7: How many ^1H NMR signals would you expect to find for the following molecules? What is the splitting pattern of each signal?

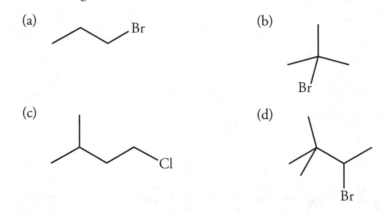

Solution:

(a) Three signals. C1's equivalent protons are split by two Hs on C2 to make a triplet. C2's protons are split by a total of five Hs on C1 and C3 to make a sextet, or multiplet. C3's protons are split by two Hs on C2 to make a triplet.

(b) One signal; all are equivalent, therefore no splitting.

(c) Four signals. C1's equivalent protons are split by two Hs on C2 to make a triplet. C2's protons are split by a total of three Hs on C1 and C3 to make a quartet. C3's proton is split by eight neighboring protons to make a multiplet. C4 and C5 have equivalent protons, split by C3's proton and forming a doublet.

(d) Three signals. The first proton signal is from the H on C3 (the one bearing the Br). It is split by three Hs on C4 to make a quartet. The Hs on C4 are split by the one H on C3 to yield a doublet. The remaining Hs on the *tert*-butyl group are equivalent (nine total), have no neighbors, and appear as a singlet.

Integration

The third important piece of information obtained from the ^1H NMR spectrum of a molecule is the mathematical integration. As the NMR instrument obtains a spectrum of the sample, it performs a mathematical calculation, called an **integration**, thereby measuring the area under each absorption peak (resonance). The calculated area under each peak is proportional to the relative number of protons giving rise to each peak. Thus, the integration indicates the relative number of protons in each set in the molecule.

The Chemical Shift

The fourth and final aspect of an NMR spectrum is the **chemical shift**, which indicates the location of the resonance (set of peaks) in the ^1H NMR spectrum. Differences in the chemical shift values for different sets of protons in a molecule are the result of the differing electronic environments that different sets of protons experience. The magnetic field created by electrons near a proton will **shield** the nucleus from the applied magnetic field created by the instrument, shifting the resonance **upfield**. The more a proton is **deshielded** (i.e., the more distorted away from the atom the electron cloud is), the further **downfield** (to the left) in an NMR spectrum it will appear. For example, a set of protons *near* an electronegative group is said to be deshielded and will appear downfield (to the left) in the ^1H NMR spectrum, relative to a set of protons that are farther away from the electronegative group, which is more shielded and appears more upfield (to the right) in the ^1H NMR spectrum.

downfield   upfield

more deshielded   less deshielded

We now briefly examine the factors involved in proton deshielding. These include:

1. the electronegativity of the neighboring atoms
2. hybridization
3. acidity and hydrogen bonding

Electronegativity Effects on Chemical Shift Values

If an electronegative atom is in close proximity to a proton, it will decrease the electron density near the proton and thereby deshield it. This will result in a *down*field shift in the chemical shift value. Examples:

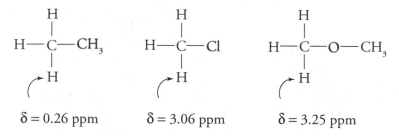

$\delta = 0.26$ ppm $\delta = 3.06$ ppm $\delta = 3.25$ ppm

The spectrum of methyl acetate below shows how the two electronegative groups in the molecule (the O of the ester and the carbonyl) contribute to shifting both methyl signals downfield.

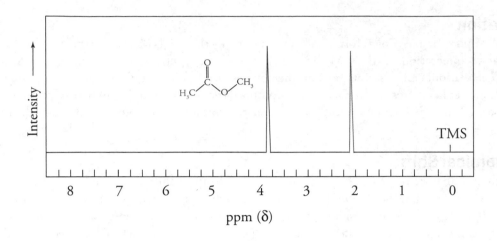

Hybridization Effects on Chemical Shift Values

The **hybridization effect** occurs as a result of the varying bond characteristics of carbon atoms *connected* to the hydrogens. The greater the *s*-orbital character of a C—H bond, the less electron density on the hydrogen. Thus, when considering the hybridization effect alone, the greater the *s*-orbital character, the more deshielded the set of protons is, which will result in a downfield shift for the peak corresponding to that set of protons. Here is an example:

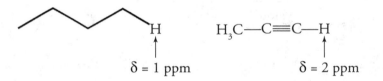

Hybridization effects alone would indicate the alkyne proton to be more deshielded than the alkene proton. However, due to a more complicated physical phenomenon, which is beyond the scope of the MCAT, this turns out not to be the case. To simplify for the MCAT, two other very characteristic chemical shifts you should be familiar with are that of the aromatic protons (δ = 6.5–8 ppm) and alkene protons (δ = 5–6 ppm).

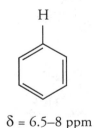

δ = 6.5–8 ppm

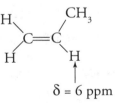

δ = 6 ppm

Acidity and Hydrogen Bonding Effects on Chemical Shift Values

Protons that are attached to **heteroatoms** (oxygen and nitrogen, for example) are quite deshielded. Acidic protons on a carboxylic acid are an extreme example of a very large downfield shift. In addition, hydrogen bonding can cause a wide variation of chemical shift. For example, the resonance of the alcohol proton in methanol varies with both solvent and temperature (different degrees of H bonding).

You should also be aware that the chemical shifts of alcohol protons are quite variable depending upon the particular compound, but are in the range of δ = 2–5 ppm.

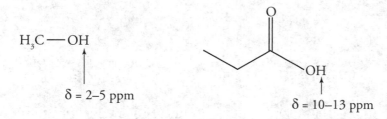

As with IR stretching frequencies, memorizing some commonly encountered ^{1}H NMR chemical shift values will be helpful. Below is a correlation chart for some common chemical shifts, the most important of which are in red:

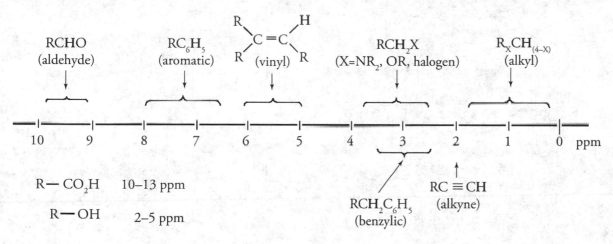

Chapter 5 Summary

- Organic compounds are separated via extraction based on their differing solubility in aqueous or organic solvents.

- Organic acids (COOHs and PhOHs) and bases (amines) can undergo acid-base reactions to generate ions, which preferentially dissolve in the aqueous layer during an extraction.

- Thin layer chromatography (TLC) separates molecules based on polarity; the more polar compound travels the least distance up the plate and has the lowest R_f value.

- Ion exchange, HPLC, size exclusion, and affinity chromatography are similar in nature to column chromatography and generally use a mobile and stationary phase for separating compounds. They are generally used to separate biomolecules like amino acids, proteins, or nucleic acids.

- Distillation and gas chromatography separate compounds based on boiling point.

- UV/Vis spectroscopy indicates the presence of a conjugated π system in a molecule, whereas IR spectroscopy identifies the functional groups present in molecules.

- The most common IR resonances tested on the MCAT are the C=O bond (≈ 1700 cm^{-1}), the C=C bond (≈ 1650 cm^{-1}) and the O—H bond (≈ 3600 cm^{-1}).

- The number of resonances in a ^{1}H NMR spectrum indicates the number of nonequivalent hydrogens present in a molecule.

- Splitting in a ^{1}H NMR spectrum occurs when one H has nonequivalent protons located on an adjacent atom (signal will be split into $n + 1$ lines; n = # of nonequivalent adjacent hydrogens).

- The number of Hs each signal represents is determined by the integration of the peak.

- Protons that are more deshielded (near electronegative groups) will be further downfield (at higher ppm), and protons that are more shielded (near electron donating groups) will be more upfield (at lower ppm).

CHAPTER 5 FREESTANDING PRACTICE QUESTIONS

1. The ^{1}H NMR spectrum for Compound X shows one peak at 7.4 ppm. If elemental analysis shows that the compound has an empirical formula of CH, how many possible stereoisomers could Compound X have?

A) 0
B) 1
C) 2
D) 4

2. How many resonances would appear in a ^{1}H NMR spectrum of the following compound?

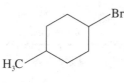

A) 3
B) 5
C) 7
D) 13

3. Consider the following reaction:

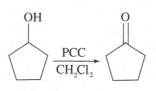

Which of the following observations about the infrared spectrum of the reaction mixture would indicate that the reaction above went to completion yielding the expected product?

A) The appearance of a stretch at 1700 cm^{-1}.
B) The disappearance of a stretch at 3300 cm^{-1}.
C) The disappearance of a stretch at 3300 cm^{-1} and the appearance of a stretch at 1700 cm^{-1}.
D) The disappearance of a stretch at 1700 cm^{-1} and the appearance of a stretch at 3300 cm^{-1}.

4. For the following reaction, how would the R_f value of the product compare to that of the starting material if monitored by TLC on a normal silica gel plate?

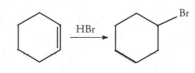

A) The R_f value of the product would be greater than that of the reactant because the product is more polar.
B) The R_f value of the product would be greater than that of the reactant because the product is less polar.
C) The R_f value of the product would be smaller than that of the reactant because the product is more polar.
D) The R_f value of the product would be smaller than that of the reactant because the product is less polar.

5. What will the ^{1}H NMR spectrum of isobutane show?

A) One 6 H triplet and one 4 H quartet
B) Two 3 H triplets and two 2 H quartets
C) One 9 H doublet and one 1 H multiplet
D) One 6 H triplet, one 2 H multiplet, and one 2 H triplet

6. Which of the following fatty acids has the highest melting point?

A) (3E, 5E)-octa-3,5-dienoic acid
B) (3E, 5E)-deca-3,5-dienoic acid
C) (3Z, 5Z)-octa-3,5-dienoic acid
D) (3Z, 5Z)-deca-3,5-dienoic acid

7. Infrared spectroscopy could be used to discern which two molecules from each other?

   I. An amine and an imine
   II. An alcohol and a carboxylic acid
   III. Glucose and fructose

A) II only
B) I and II only
C) I and III only
D) I, II, and III

CHAPTER 5 PRACTICE PASSAGE

13-Deoxytetrodecamycin (1) was isolated from WAC04657, a wild-isolate *Streptomyces* that has antibiotic activities against drug resistant Gram-negative and Gram-positive pathogens. 13-Deoxytetrodecamycin is a congener of the tetrodecamycin family (Figure 1), lacking the *trans* hydroxyl on C-13 on the decalin type ring system, and all molecules possess some antimicrobial activity. 13-Deoxytetrodecamycin was isolated as a white residue and is soluble in DMSO and $CHCl_3$. It has a molecular formula of $C_{18}H_{22}O_5$, and its exact mass was found via high-resolution mass spectrometry as the sodium complex.

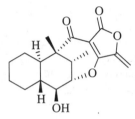

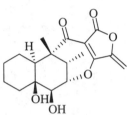

13-deoxytetrodecamycin (1)   tetrodecamycin (2)

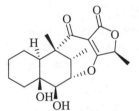

dihydrotetrodecamycin (3)

Figure 1   Tetrodecamycin family of molecules

In order to isolate the compounds associated with the bioactivity, solid agar cultures of WAC04657 were grown and extracted with ethyl acetate. The ethyl acetate was concentrated, and the crude extract was dissolved in chloroform. The extracts were separated by TLC, and the plates were overlaid with the bacterium *Bacillus subtilis*. In order to analyze the plate, the cells were stained with thiazolyl blue tetrazolium bromide (MTT), after which, the appropriate band of silica was extracted with chloroform and subjected to reverse-phase HPLC analysis. The chromatograph revealed that the band of silica consisted of one primary peak (Figure 2). This peak was determined to be 1. The semi-pure product was used to develop an HPLC purification of the compound from large-scale crude extracts (Figure 3).

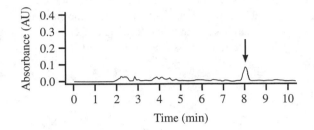

Figure 2   HPLC trace of TLC purified compound

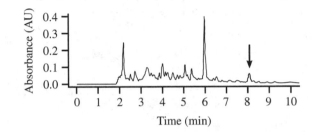

Figure 3   HPLC trace of crude extract

In order to sufficiently study the bioactivity of **1**, a large-scale isolation and purification procedure was developed. The solid MYM agar (12.8 L) was macerated and extracted with an equal volume of ethyl acetate. The ethyl acetate was filtered and concentrated under vacuum giving a brown extract. The extract was suspended in 50% H_2O/acetonitrile and loaded onto a Sep-Pak C18 column. The column was washed with 10 mL each of H_2O and 30% aqueous acetonitrile, then the desired compound was eluted with 70% aqueous acetonitrile. The solvent was evaporated and redissolved in 50% aqueous acetonitrile. After two HPLC purifications, 1.1 mg of pure **1** was isolated as a white residue.

(Adapted from Gverzdys, T.; Hart. M. K.; Pimentel-Elardo, S.; Tranmer, G.; Nodwell, J. R. *J. Antibiot. (Tokyo)*, 2010, *63*, 1.)

1. Mitochondrial dehydrogenase in living cells converts the yellow dye MTT, commonly used in cell proliferation assays, into MTT-formazan, which is purple in color. What feature(s) of the TLC plate would allow for the isolation of the appropriate compound from the silica gel?

A) The TLC plate would be white and the appropriate band would be purple.
B) The TLC plate would be yellow and the appropriate band would be purple.
C) The TLC plate would be purple and the appropriate band would be white.
D) The TLC plate would be purple and the appropriate band would be yellow.

2. What *m/z* value was experimentally determined in the isolation of 13-deoxytetrodecamycin?

A) 317
B) 341
C) 340
D) 319

3. Both 13-deoxytetrodecamycin and the C-14 epimer of tetrodecamycin were independently reacted with *p*-toluenesulfonyl chloride (TsCl) in the presence of base, and each gave distinct products. Which of the following steps is LEAST likely to occur in either mechanism of the reactions?

A) TsCl will react with the alcohol of 13-deoxytetrodecamycin to generate a good leaving group, which will eliminate at C-13 to yield an alkene.
B) TsCl will react with the secondary alcohol of the C-14 epimer of tetrodecamycin to generate a good leaving group, which the C-13 hydroxyl will displace to yield an epoxide.
C) TsCl will react with the tertiary alcohol of the C-14 epimer of tetrodecamycin to generate a good leaving group, which the C-14 hydroxyl will displace to yield an epoxide.
D) TsCl will react with the alcohol of 13-deoxytetrodecamycin to generate a good leaving group, which can leave to yield a carbocation intermediate.

4. Supercritical fluid chromatography (SFC) uses supercritical fluid CO_2 in the mobile phase, and like HPLC, both normal and ODS(C18)-packed columns can be used. If the crude extract in the passage was purified by SFC using a C-18 column, how would the analysis chromatogram for the separation of the indicated product compare to Figure 3?

A) The desired product would have a longer retention time because CO_2 is a nonpolar solvent.
B) The desired product would have a similar retention time because both purifications use a reverse-phase column.
C) The desired product would have a similar retention time because the column is irrelevant in stationary-mobile phase chromatography.
D) The desired product would have a shorter retention time because CO_2 is a polar solvent.

5. Which of the following describes the configuration at C-14 in 13-deoxy-14-*epi*-tetrodecamycin and the position of its OH group?

A) *R*, axial
B) *R*, equatorial
C) *S*, axial
D) *S*, equatorial

SOLUTIONS TO CHAPTER 5 FREESTANDING PRACTICE QUESTIONS

1. **A** One signal on the ^{1}H NMR spectrum tells us that the molecule has only one type of hydrogen. Since the empirical formula of Compound X is CH and the molecule contains no electronegative elements to shift the signal downfield, the single peak, located in the region common for aromatic hydrogens (7–8 ppm), must represent an aromatic H. Any compound with only aromatic Hs must have carbons that are all sp^2 hybridized, and as such will have no stereoisomers. In this case, the compound is benzene (C_6H_6).

2. **B** By showing the hydrogens, one would expect the molecule to have five resonances in a ^{1}H NMR spectrum. Note the plane of symmetry through the molecule (as shown with the dotted line). Both sets of CH_2 hydrogens on the carbons adjacent to the bromo and methyl substituents are chemically equivalent to each other.

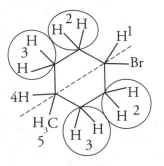

3. **C** The reaction is a transformation from an alcohol to a ketone. In an infrared spectrum, this can be noticed by the disappearance of the broad O—H stretch around 3300 cm^{-1}, and the appearance of the C=O stretch at 1700 cm^{-1}. Choices A and B are incorrect because the appearance of the C=O stretch does not automatically translate that the oxidation reaction went to completion and the disappearance of the O—H stretch doesn't mean that the desired product is formed. In order for the reaction to be complete, one must disappear as the other appears. Choice D is incorrect as the stretches that would appear and disappear are incorrect for the corresponding functional group transformation.

4. **C** TLC separates compounds based on their polarities. The more polar a compound is, the more it adheres to the silica gel plate, giving it a smaller R_f value. Choices A and D are inconsistent with this type of interaction. The product for this reaction is bromocyclohexane, which is more polar than the reactant due to the presence of the halogen.

5. **C** The structure of isobutane is shown below. All three terminal CH_3 groups are chemically identical, and will show up as one resonance. More specifically, they will correspond to a doublet as they are split by the sole proton on the central carbon. The proton on the central carbon will show up as a multiplet, as it is split by 9 equivalent H atoms. Thus, one 9 H doublet and one 1 H multiplet is the correct answer.

6. **B** In general, larger molecules have higher melting points due to increased London dispersion forces. Eliminate choices A and C since they have eight carbons (octa), while the molecules in choices B and D have ten carbons (deca). The remaining difference between B and D is the presence of *E* or *Z* double bonds. *Z* double bonds introduce kinks in the fatty acid chain, making it more difficult for the molecules to pack together, therefore reducing their melting point. This eliminates choice D.

7. **B** Infrared spectroscopy identifies functional groups. Since all Roman numeral items refer to molecules with different functional groups, choice D is a tempting answer. Item I refers to a molecule with a C—N bond (amine) and a molecule with a C=N bond (imine) which will generate different resonances. Since Item I is true, choice A can be eliminated. Item II compares an alcohol with an –OH group to a carboxyl group (–COOH). While this compound will have an –OH signal in its spectrum, it will also have a peak for the carbonyl making it distinguishable from the alcohol. Since Item II is true, choice C can be eliminated. However, Item III is false, because even though glucose is an aldose (contains an aldehyde), these functional groups both have the C=O bond and their possible regions in the IR spectrum overlap. Thus these molecules would be difficult to distinguish using infrared spectroscopy, making choice B the correct answer.

SOLUTIONS TO CHAPTER 5 PRACTICE PASSAGE

1. **D** The TLC plate in the passage is overlaid with *Bacillus subtilis*, which possess the cellular activity to reduce the yellow MTT to purple MTT-formazan. Thus the plate will have a purple color (eliminate choices A and B). Since the TLC plate is separating the molecules that are active against *Bacillus subtilis*, the bands of silica at the R_f values for those molecules will not have microbial growth. With no cellular activity, those bands will remain yellow, the color of MTT (choice D is correct).

2. **B** The passage states that 13-deoxytetrodecamycin has a molecular formula of $C_{18}H_{22}O_5$ and that the exact mass was experimentally found as the sodium complex. The molar mass of 13-deoxytetrodecamycin is 318 g/mol, and sodium has a molar mass of ~23 g/mol, giving 318 + 23 = 341 (choice B is correct).

3. **C** In the presence of TsCl and base, 13-deoxytetrodecamycin should generate an alkene between C-13 and C-14 via a carbocation intermediate (eliminate choices A and D), while the C-14 epimer of tetrodecamycin should produce an epoxide between carbons C-13 and C-14 (via an S_N2-like reaction) as the answer choices suggest. However, in both reactions the secondary alcohol will be activated with the tosyl group, as it's the least sterically hindered alcohol. Therefore, choice C is the correct answer, as the tertiary alcohol will NOT get activated as the leaving group.

4. **B**   SFC uses supercritical fluid CO_2 as a nonpolar solvent for the separation of compounds (eliminate choice D). As the question states, it can use both normal and C-18 columns, and regardless of normal or reverse phase, the column is critical for separating polar and nonpolar compounds (eliminate choice C). Finally since the purification is occurring on a stationary phase similar to that in Figure 3, the retention time of the indicated product purified by SFC would be similar to that of Figure 3 (eliminate choice A). Therefore, choice B is the correct answer.

5. **A**   13-Deoxy-14-*epi*-tetrodecamycin is the C-14 epimer of compound 1. The figure below shows the appropriate prioritization of the four groups attached to C-14:

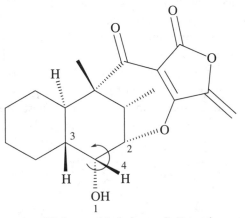

13-deoxy-14- epi-tetrodecamycin

The OH group has the highest priority because oxygen has the highest atomic number of the four groups, and hydrogen is the lowest priority as it has the lowest atomic number. The remaining priority assignments are between two carbon substituents, so we must find the first point of difference. C-13 (at the ring juncture) is bonded to two other carbons, while the final substituent is bonded to a carbon and an oxygen. Since the oxygen has the higher atomic number, the carbon on the right gets the higher priority when compared to C-13. When the arc from 1 → 2 → 3 is traced in a counterclockwise direction, since the lowest priority group is oriented in front of the molecule instead of in the back, we must choose the opposite configuration than what we'd expect, making the configuration *R* (eliminate choices C and D).

13-Deoxy-14-*epi*-tetrodecamycin has a *trans*-fused decalin ring system, making the hydrogens on the fused carbons axial. This is the case for all *trans*-fused decalins, since if the hydrogens were equatorial, the fused ring would have to adopt an impossible geometry (see figure below) in order to make a six-membered ring.

trans-decalin

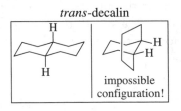

Since the C-13 hydrogen is axial and is in the up configuration, the down configuration on C-14 (which is where the OH group is) will also be axial, making choice A the correct answer.

Chapter 6
Carbonyl Chemistry

In this chapter we will discuss the major reaction types: nucleophilic substitution and addition. Each reaction type is defined by the bonding changes that occur over the course of the reaction.

In a substitution reaction, one σ bond in the starting material is converted into a new σ bond in the product. We will briefly explore the two most common substitution reactions.

In an addition reaction, one π bond in the starting material is converted into 2 new σ bonds in the product. Addition will be the principal focus of this chapter as it relates to the carbonyl functional group, a group that appears in all major biomolecules. In addition to this reactivity, carbonyl-containing compounds will undergo deprotonation of the α-carbon atom. We will learn in this chapter how these two reactivities interrelate.

6.1 NUCLEOPHILIC SUBSTITUTIONS

Nucleophilic substitution reactions replace a leaving group in an electrophilic substrate with a nucleophile. In this context, the bonds that break during the substitution will do so via a heterolytic cleavage where the leaving group takes both electrons from the bond that connected it to the electrophile. This also means you can recognize a substitution reaction by the fact that one σ bond is broken to the leaving group while another is formed to the incoming nucleophile. Therefore, there is no net change in the number of σ bonds or π bonds over the course of the reaction.

Before you read on about the two main nucleophilic substitution mechanisms—S_N1 and S_N2—go back to the Organic Chemist's Toolbox in Section 4.1 to review the three main players involved in all nucleophilic substitution reactions: nucleophiles, electrophiles, and leaving groups.

The S_N2 Mechanism

The first nucleophilic mechanism we'll examine is the S_N2 mechanism. Typical electrophiles (also known as the substrates) for this type of reaction are alkyl halides. Alkyl halides are alkanes that contain at least one halogen (fluorine, chlorine, bromine or iodine). Since halogen atoms are electronegative, are large in size, and are the conjugate bases of strong acids (except for F^-), most halides (Cl^-, Br^-, I^-) make good leaving groups.

For example, when 1-iodobutane is treated with a Br^- nucleophile, an S_N2 reaction occurs in which bromide replaces the I^- group (known as the leaving group) to yield 1-bromobutane.

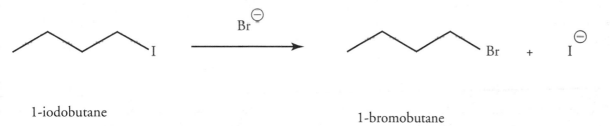

1-iodobutane

1-bromobutane

In the first (and only) step of this reaction (see the mechanism below), because the nucleophilic bromide anion attacks the electrophilic carbon at the *same time* that the leaving group leaves, the attack must occur *from the backside* of the substrate. The bromine-carbon bond forms as the iodine-carbon bond is broken, *in a single step*, to yield bromobutane.

The Mechanism

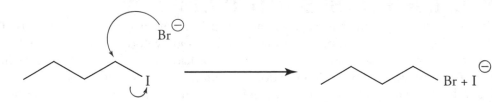

Let's look at a chiral substrate in order to see the stereochemical implications of this concerted mechanism. When (*R*)-1-deutero-1-chloroethane is treated with iodide, the typical backside attack occurs. As the new C—I bond begins to form while the C—Cl bond breaks, the reaction proceeds through a *pentavalent transition state*. As you can see in the product below, there is complete *inversion of configuration* at the carbon being attacked by the nucleophile. This is always the case in an S$_N$2 reaction on a chiral substrate.

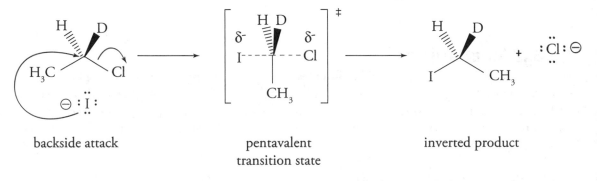

| backside attack | pentavalent transition state | inverted product |

Furthermore, the rate of the reaction is a function of two variables—that is, **bimolecular**. The rate of the reaction depends on the concentrations of both the nucleophile and the electrophile, and is equal to the product of the rate constant (*k*), the concentration of the nucleophile ([I$^-$]), and the concentration of the electrophile ([R-Cl]).

$$\text{reaction rate} = k[\text{nucleophile}][\text{electrophile}]$$

We can now explain what we mean when we say that this reaction proceeds by an "S$_N$2" mechanism. The "S" indicates that it is a <u>s</u>ubstitution reaction mechanism, the subscript "N" indicates that it is <u>n</u>ucleophilic, and the "2" indicates that it is <u>b</u>imolecular (see General Chemistry Review Section 9.4 for more details on rate laws).

The rate of the reaction depends not only on the concentration of the electrophile, but also on the degree of substitution of the electrophilic carbon. Since the transition state is sterically crowded with five groups attached, the more bulky those groups are, the harder it is for the nucleophile to gain access to the reactive site. Therefore, less substituted substrates react faster than more substituted ones via the S$_N$2 mechanism.

The last factor to consider in substitution reactions is the solvent. To favor an S$_N$2 mechanism, protic solvents such as water and alcohols should be avoided. Since these hydrogen bonding solvents are able to strongly solvate the nucleophile, they hinder the backside attack necessary for the concerted reaction. To prevent this interference, polar, *aprotic* solvents such as acetone, DMF (dimethylformamide), or DMSO (dimethylsulfoxide) should be used. Their polar nature allows the charged nucleophiles and leaving groups to remain dissolved, but they are not as efficient at completely solvating the nucleophile.

Key Features of an S$_N$2 Reaction

Reactivity of substrate: CH_3 > 1° > 2° >> 3°   (Because of steric hindrance)

Stereochemistry: Complete stereochemical inversion of the carbon that is attacked by the nucleophile.

Kinetics: reaction rate = k[nucleophile][electrophile]

Solvent: S$_N$2 reactions are favored by polar, aprotic (non-hydrogen bonding) solvents.

Rearrangements: Not possible due to concerted mechanism. No carbocations are present in solution.

Favoring Conditions: Strong, non-bulky nucleophile will favor S$_N$2 reactions over S$_N$1 (see next section).

The S$_N$1 Mechanism

In contrast to the concerted S$_N$2 mechanism, the course of S$_N$1 substitution reactions, a carbocation (carbonium ion) forms. Let's take a moment to review the relative stability of carbocations. Remember that the formation of charged species from neutral ones is generally an energetically disfavorable process; that is, it is energetically *uphill*. But some ions are more stable than others. For alkyl cations, the relative stabilities due to the inductive effect (Section 4.1) are given below.

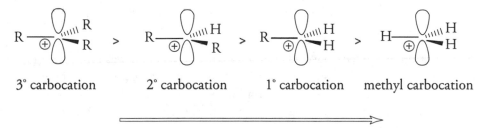

3° carbocation   2° carbocation   1° carbocation   methyl carbocation

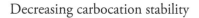

Decreasing carbocation stability

Now that we have reviewed the basics of carbocation stability, let's consider an example where a chiral halide undergoes an S$_N$1 substitution reaction. When (*R*)-3-bromo-3-methylhexane is treated with H$_2$O, a racemic mixture of 3-methylhexan-3-ol is formed:

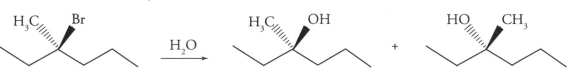

(*R*)-3-bromo-3-methylhexane   (*R*)-3-methylhexan-3-ol   (*S*)-3-methylhexan-3-ol

S_N1 substitution occurs in *two distinct steps*, unlike S_N2 reactions that occur in one step. In the first step of the S_N1 reaction, a *planar carbocation* with 120° bond angles forms (see mechanism below). This occurs when the leaving group falls off (dissociates). This is the slow step of the mechanism, or the rate limiting step. In the final step of this reaction, *racemization* occurs as the nucleophile attacks equally *on either side* of the carbocation. The result is a racemic mixture.

The Mechanism

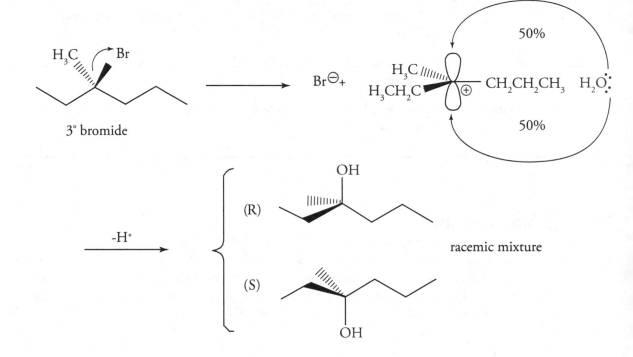

Unlike the S_N2 reaction explained above where the rate of the reaction was a function of two variables, the S_N1 reaction rate is a function of only one variable, that is, **unimolecular**. The rate of the S_N1 reaction depends only upon the concentration of the electrophile (the species that loses the leaving group over the course of the reaction). The rate of the reaction is equal to the product of the rate constant (k), and the electrophile concentration ([R-Br]):

$$\text{reaction rate} = k[\text{electrophile}]$$

As before, we can now explain what we mean when we say that this reaction proceeds by an "S_N1" mechanism. The "S" indicates that it is a <u>s</u>ubstitution reaction mechanism, the subscript "N" indicates that it is <u>n</u>ucleophic, and the "1" indicates that it is <u>uni</u>molecular.

The rate of the reaction depends not only on the concentration of the electrophile, but also on the degree of substitution of the electrophilic carbon. Since the dissociation of the leaving group is the slow step of the mechanism, anything that makes that step more favorable will speed up the reaction. As was just discussed, the more substituted the carbocation intermediate, the more stable it is. Therefore, more substituted substrates will dissociate to make more stable intermediates faster, speeding up the rate of the entire reaction.

To favor an S_N1 mechanism, protic solvents such as water and alcohols should be used. The role of the solvent is twofold. The protic solvent helps to stabilize the forming carbocation and solvate the leaving group, thereby facilitating the first, or slow step of the mechanism. Secondly, the solvent then behaves as the nucleophile in a **solvolysis** reaction, attacking the carbocation intermediate. This produces an alcohol product if water is used as the solvent and an ether if the reaction is run in an alcoholic solvent.

Key Features of an S_N1 Reaction

Reactivity of substrate:	$3° > 2° \gg 1°$ (Due to stabilization of the carbocation.)
Stereochemistry:	Almost complete racemization due to nucleophilic attack on either side of p orbital.
Kinetics:	reaction rate = k[electrophile]
Solvent:	S_N1 reactions are favored by protic (hydrogen bonding) solvents. (This stabilizes the carbocation.)
Rearrangements:	Carbocation rearrangement is possible; if the carbocation can rearrange to one that is more stable, it will.
Favoring conditions:	Non-basic, weaker nucleophiles favor unimolecular substitutions.

Alcohols undergo substitution reactions just as alkyl halides do. They can undergo either S_N1 or S_N2 substitution reactions depending upon the degree of substitution of the alcohol. Alcohols are treated with strong mineral acids to make their bad –OH leaving group into a good one (H_2O). In S_N2 reactions, the conjugate base of the mineral acid will attack while the leaving group leaves. In S_N1 reactions, the water will first dissociate, followed by nucleophilic attack of the halide ion on the carbocation intermediate.

Example 6-1: Predict whether the following substitution reactions will proceed via an S_N1 or an S_N2 mechanism.

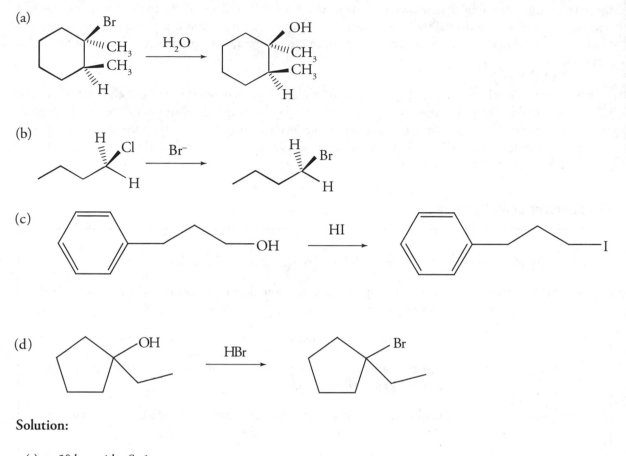

Solution:

(a) 3° bromide, S_N1
(b) 1° chloride, S_N2
(c) 1° alcohol, S_N2
(d) 3° alcohol, S_N1

6.2 ALDEHYDES AND KETONES

Two very important classes of oxygen-containing organic compounds are aldehydes and ketones. We begin the discussion of these functional groups by looking at a common way carbonyls are formed—the oxidation of an alcohol:

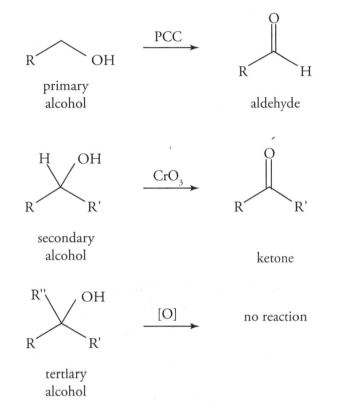

Note: Since the oxidizing agent removes a hydrogen from the carbon, tertiary alcohols are not able to react to form carbonyls since they have no hydrogen at the reactive site.

Oxidizing agents are able to absorb electrons (and be reduced). Below are some common oxidizing agents that appear on the MCAT. Note that only the anhydrous oxidant (PCC) will NOT overoxidize the primary alcohol to the carboxylic acid (we'll talk more about this functional group later). All oxidizing agents shown can be used to form ketones from secondary alcohols.

Aqueous Oxidants	Anhydrous Oxidant
Chromic Acid (H_2CrO_4)	
Chromate Salts (CrO_4^{2-})	
Dichromate Salts ($Cr_2O_7^{2-}$)	Pyridinium Chlorochromate (PCC)
Permanganate (MnO_4^-)	
Chromium Trioxide (CrO_3)	

Now that we understand how aldehydes and ketones are formed, let's look at their reactivities. The key to understanding the chemistry of aldehydes and ketones is to understand the electronic structure and properties of the carbonyl group. The C=O double bond is very polarized because oxygen is much more electronegative than carbon, and so it is able to pull the π electrons of the C=O double bond toward itself and away from carbon. This is illustrated by the following resonance structures:

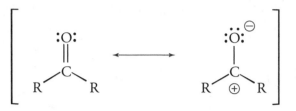

So overall, carbonyls react like

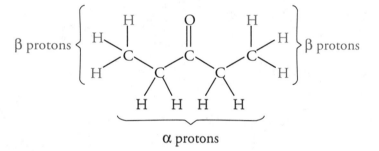

This bond polarization renders the carbon atom electrophilic (δ^+) and accounts for two kinds of reactions of aldehydes and ketones. First, these molecules have *acidic protons α to (i.e., next to) the carbonyl group.*

An α-proton is acidic because the electrons left behind upon deprotonation can delocalize into the π system of the carbonyl. Second, the electrophilic carbon of the carbonyl group makes aldehydes and ketones *susceptible to nucleophilic attack*. In the aldol condensation, which we will study in some detail, both of these types of reactivity are involved in a single reaction.

Acidity and Enolization

The first type of reaction that is commonly observed with aldehydes and ketones is the result of the relative acidity of protons that are α to the carbonyl group. These α-protons are sufficiently acidic that they can be removed by a strong base [such as hydroxide ion (OH⁻) or an alkoxide ion (OR⁻)] to yield a carbanion. This carbanion can be easily formed because the electrons that are left behind on the carbon can be delocalized into the carbonyl π system. In this way, the negative charge can be delocalized onto the electronegative oxygen atom. A resonance-stabilized carbanion of this type is referred to as an **enolate ion**. *An enolate ion* *is negatively charged and nucleophilic.* The nucleophilic character of an enolate ion lies predominantly at the carbon at which the proton was abstracted, *not* the oxygen atom of the carbonyl. This is why the α-carbon of enolates is the nucleophile in most common enolate reactions.

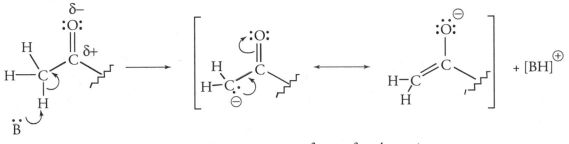

resonance forms of enolate anion

An example that demonstrates the acidity of α-protons is the exchange reaction that occurs between the α-proton of Compound I (below) and deuterium from D_2O. Compound I has a single α-proton that is α to *two* carbonyl groups in comparison to the six other α-protons in the molecule that are α to only *one* carbonyl group. It is this lone α-proton that exchanges with a deuterium of D_2O over the course of a couple of days, even in the absence of base. Being next to two carbonyl groups greatly enhances the acidity of this α-proton and allows it to exchange (although slowly) with a deuterium from D_2O. The mechanism of this exchange, which essentially consists of protonation of the intermediate enolate ion, is shown in the following figure:

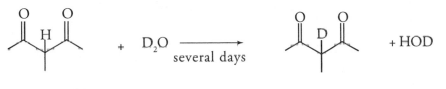

Compound I

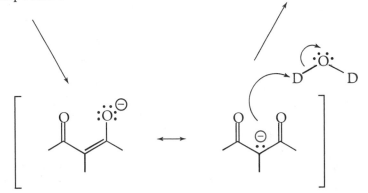

Example 6-2: As a review of acidity, for each of the following pairs of compounds, identify the one with the more acidic proton.

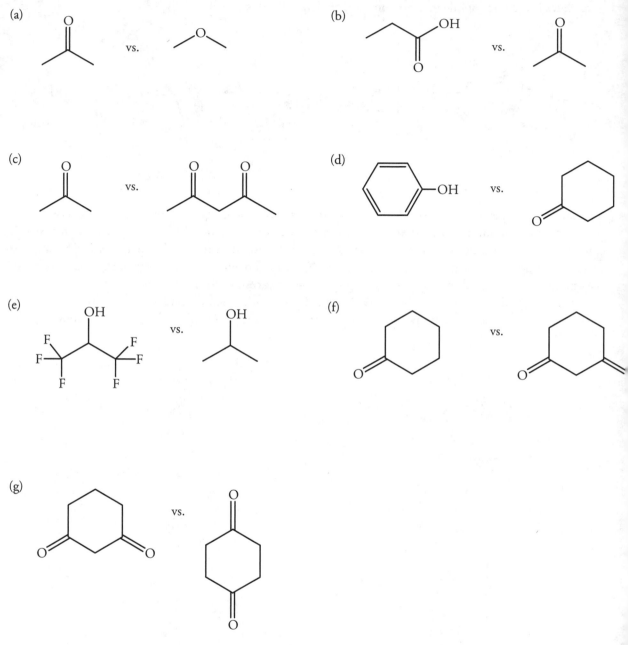

Solution:

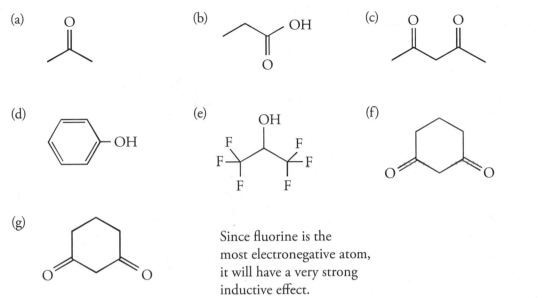

(g)

Since fluorine is the
most electronegative atom,
it will have a very strong
inductive effect.

Keto-Enol Tautomerism

A ketone is converted into an enol by deprotonation of an α-carbon atom and subsequent protonation of
the carbonyl oxygen. These two forms of the molecule are very similar to one another and differ only by
the position of a proton and a double bond. This is referred to as **keto-enol tautomerism**. Two molecules
are **tautomers** if they are readily interconvertible constitutional isomers in equilibrium with one another.

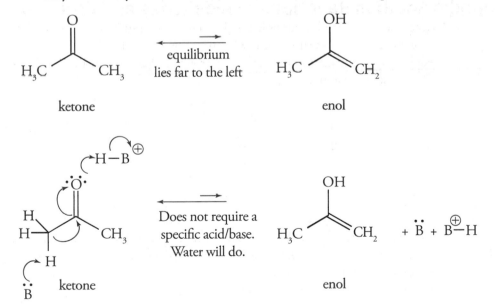

Tautomerization has consequences for molecules with chiral α-carbons. Imagine an alcohol with a chiral center adjacent to the hydroxyl group (as shown below). If this stereochemically-defined alcohol were oxidized, the corresponding ketone would have racemic stereochemistry.

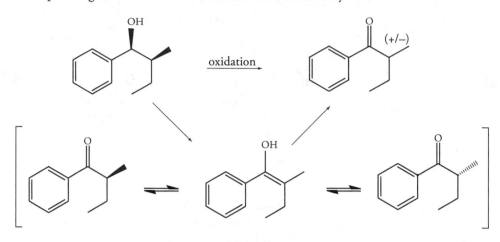

Because the α-carbon of the compound is sp^2 hybridized and planar in the enol tautomer, protonation to form the keto tautomer can occur from both the top and bottom faces of the double bond. This loss of defined stereochemistry, which results in a mixture of *R* and *S* configurations at the once chiral α-carbon, is termed **racemization**.

Nucleophilic Addition Reactions to Aldehydes and Ketones

Because of the polarized nature of the C=O double bond in aldehydes and ketones, the carbon of the carbonyl group is very electrophilic. This means that it will attract nucleophiles and can readily be reduced. The attack of a nucleophile upon the carbon of a carbonyl group, called a nucleophilic addition reaction, is shown below with a generic nucleophile (Nu:).

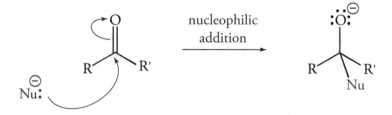

Nucleophilic addition reactions are defined by the bonding changes that occur over the course of the reaction. In these reactions, a π bond in the starting material is broken, and two σ bonds in the product result. This very general reaction allows for the conversion of aldehydes or ketones into a variety of other functional groups, such as alcohols, via hydride reduction:

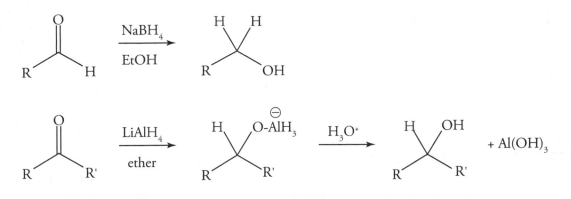

Note: Sodium borohydride ($NaBH_4$) and lithium aluminum hydride ($LiAlH_4$) are common reducing agents seen on the MCAT. In general, strong reducing agents easily lose electrons by adding hydride (a hydrogen atom and a pair of electrons) to the carbonyl. Reducing agents often have many hydrogens attached to other elements with low electronegativity.

Organometallic Reagents

Organometallic reagents are commonly used to perform nucleophilic addition to a carbonyl carbon. The basic structure of an organometallic reagent is R^-M^+. They act as electron rich, or anionic carbon atoms and therefore function as either strong bases or nucleophiles. Grignard and lithium reagents are the most common organometallic reagents.

Grignard reagents are generally made via the action of an alkyl or acyl halide on magnesium metal, as depicted below.

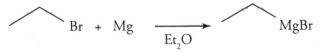

To avoid unwanted protonation of the very basic Grignard reagent, the reaction is carried out in an aprotic solvent such as diethyl ether.

The carbonyl containing compounds are then added to the Grignard reagents to yield alcohol products. In the reaction below, the methyl magnesium bromide acts as a nucleophile and adds to the electrophilic carbonyl carbon. An intermediate alkoxide ion is formed that is rapidly protonated to produce the alcohol during an aqueous acidic workup step.

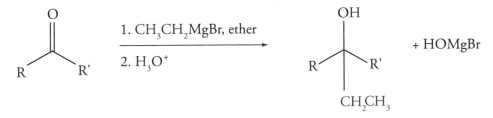

In addition to using an aprotic solvent, care must also be taken to avoid the presence of any other acidic hydrogens in the substrate molecule bearing the carbonyl. This means that alcohol groups or carboxylic acid groups must be absent, or else first be protected, before the Grignard reagent can be added to the carbonyl compound.

Mesylates and Tosylates

Two commonly used strategies for the protection of alcohols are their transformation into mesylates and tosylates. By adding a mesyl (methanesulfonyl, $CH_3-SO_3^-$) or tosyl group (toluenesulfonyl, $CH_3C_6H_4-SO_3^-$) in the place of hydroxyl, the reactive nature of the protic, and potentially nucleophilic –OH group is removed, allowing the molecule to participate in reactions the presence of the hydroxyl may have prevented.

The formation of mesylates and tosylates from alcohols are shown below. Reaction of a sulfonyl chloride, either mesyl chloride or tosyl chloride, with an alcohol in the presence of a base (generally triethylamine or pyridine) leads to nucleophilic attack at the sulfur, followed by expulsion of the chloride.

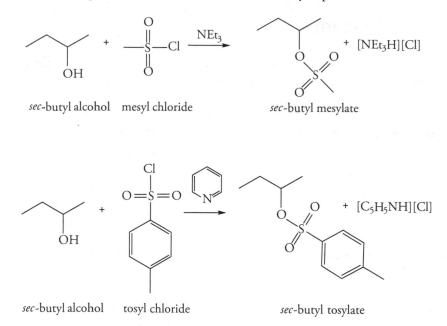

sec-butyl alcohol	mesyl chloride	*sec*-butyl mesylate

sec-butyl alcohol	tosyl chloride	*sec*-butyl tosylate

The base in each reaction is required to neutralize the HCl (consisting of the hydroxyl proton and the chloride from the sulfonyl group) and pull it out of solution as an ammonium or pyridinium chloride salt.

These groups, particularly the tosyl group, may be similarly utilized in the protection of amino ($-NH_2$) groups. In either case, hydroxyl or amino, the protected functionality is rendered sufficiently inert for the purposes of the subsequent reaction steps. Once the protection is no longer required, the protecting group may be removed and the hydroxyl or amine functionality regenerated, generally under reductive conditions.

In addition to their use as protecting groups, both mesylates and tosylates are good leaving groups in reactions featuring nucleophilic attack. Whereas hydroxyl is a poor leaving group requiring a very strong nucleophile for displacement, conversion of a hydroxyl into a mesylate or tosylate makes attack and displacement facile.

Acetals and Hemiacetals

Acetals and hemiacetals, which are of fundamental importance in biochemical reactions that occur in living organisms, can be synthesized from nucleophilic addition reactions to aldehydes or ketones. There are many examples of these molecules in common biochemical pathways. Before we learn the chemistry of these groups, we must be able to identify acetals and hemiacetals.

Note: The terms *ketal* and *hemiketal* refer to acetals and hemiacetals made from *ketones*, but this nomenclature appears infrequently.

General Formulas

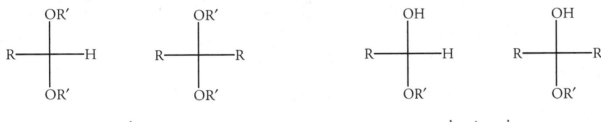

acetals   hemiacetals

Some Specific Examples

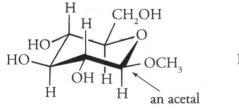

an acetal

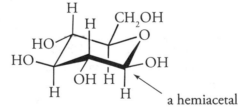

a hemiacetal

Example 6-3: For each of the following compounds, identify whether it's an acetal, hemiacetal, or neither:

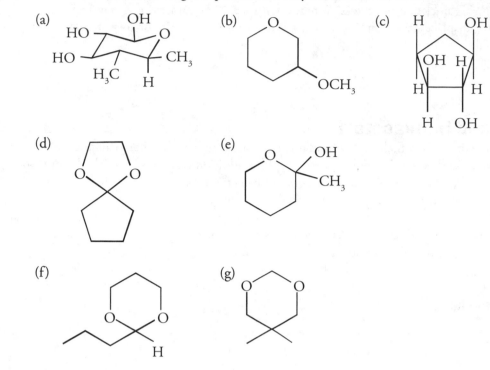

Solution:

(a) hemiacetal
(b) neither
(c) neither
(d) acetal
(e) hemiacetal
(f) acetal
(g) acetal

Acetals are formed when aldehydes or ketones react with alcohols in the presence of acid. This occurs by a nucleophilic addition mechanism. It is easy to predict the product of an acetal formation reaction. Notice that *hydrogens or carbons attached to the carbonyl carbon* of the aldehyde or ketone *remain attached* in the acetal product with the subsequent addition of two –OR groups from the alcohol. Also, note that an intermediate hemiacetal results from the addition of one –OR group to an aldehyde or ketone with subsequent protonation of the carbonyl oxygen. The aldehyde or ketone, the hemiacetal, and the acetal are all in equilibrium with one another. In order for the hemiacetal to form the acetal, a molecule of water must be lost.

Acetal Formation

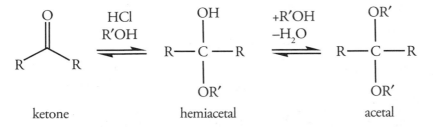

ketone   hemiacetal   acetal

The mechanism of this important reaction is shown below. In the first step, the carbonyl oxygen is protonated, making the carbonyl carbon even more susceptible to nucleophilic attack by the oxygen of the attacking alcohol molecule. Following nucleophilic attack, the oxygen of the alcohol nucleophile is positively charged. This positive charge is unfavorable, and neutrality is achieved by loss of a proton, which yields the intermediate hemiacetal. Remember that the reaction mixture is acidic so that a lone pair of electrons on the hemiacetal –OH can be protonated, thereby converting a poor leaving group into a good leaving group. Once again, this increases the electrophilicity of the carbon and makes it more susceptible to a second nucleophilic attack by an alcohol molecule. All that remains is for the positively charged oxygen from the attacking alcohol to lose a proton to yield the acetal product.

The Mechanism

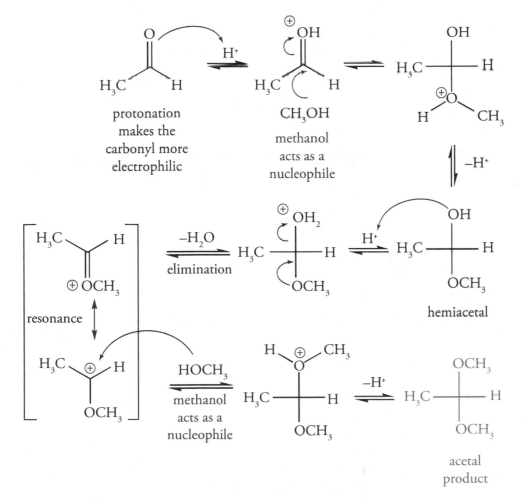

The Overall Reaction

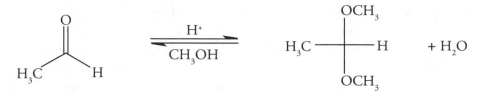

Example 6-4: Predict the acetal product from the following reactions:

(a)

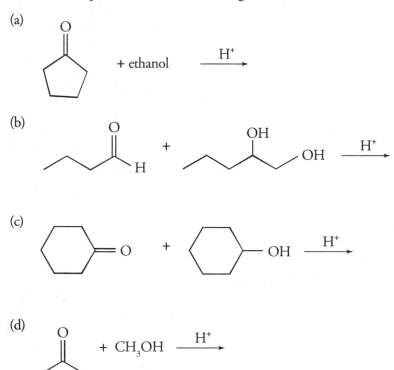

(b)

(c)

(d)

Solution:

(a) C_2H_5O OC_2H_5

(b)

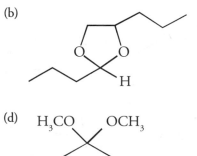

(c)

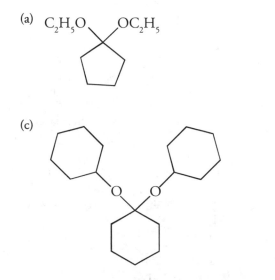

(d) H_3CO OCH_3

Cyanohydrin Formation

Whereas the nucleophilic attack of an alcohol or alkoxide on a ketone or aldehyde leads to the formation of a tetrahedral hemiacetal, attack by cyanide ($^-$C≡N) results in the formation of a cyanohydrin. The mechanism, shown below, is very similar to the one at work in the formation of hemiacetals. While cyanohydrin formation can be technically envisioned as an equilibrium process, much like the formation of hemiacetals, the equilibrium heavily favors the products and can practically be envisioned as a one-way reaction.

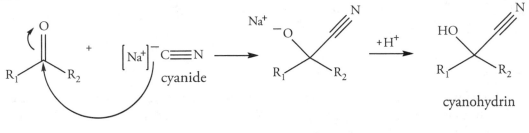

cyanohydrin

Amines

Before looking at the next few examples of nucleophilic addition reactions, we should first briefly discuss the nucleophile used in the reactions—namely amines. Organic compounds that contain nitrogen are of fundamental importance in biological systems. The most common class of nitrogen-containing compounds are referred to as **amines** and have the general structure of R–NH$_2$. Amines can be further classified as either **alkyl amines** or **aryl amines**. *Alkyl* amines are compounds in which nitrogen is bound to an sp^3-hybridized carbon, while *aryl* amines are compounds in which nitrogen is bonded to an sp^2-hybridized carbon of an aromatic ring.

Below are a few examples of common amines.

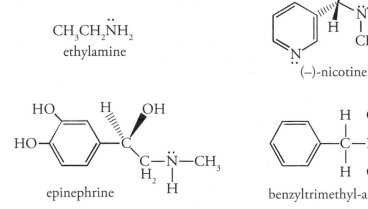

CH$_3$CH$_2$NH$_2$
ethylamine

(−)-nicotine

epinephrine

benzyltrimethyl-ammonium chloride

6.2

Amines can be further categorized as primary amines, secondary amines, tertiary amines, and quaternary ammonium ions.

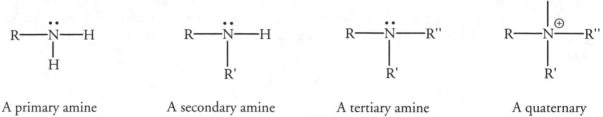

A primary amine   A secondary amine   A tertiary amine   A quaternary
ammonium ion

In the simple methyl amine, CH_3NH_2, notice that the nitrogen has three σ bonds and one lone electron pair. Its hybridization is therefore sp^3 with approximately 109° bond angles. The molecular geometry of an alkyl amine is pyramidal.

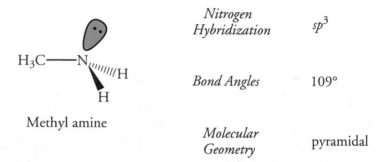

Methyl amine

Nitrogen Hybridization	sp^3
Bond Angles	109°
Molecular Geometry	pyramidal

Most importantly, because of the lone pair of electrons on the N, amines behave as either Brønsted-Lowry bases or as nucleophiles. Let's now look at a few reactions in which the nucleophile is an amine.

Imine Formation

A class of reactions that closely resembles acetal formation are the reactions of aldehydes or ketones with amines. These reactions are often catalyzed under weakly acidic conditions (pH about 4-5). When an aldehyde or ketone reacts with a primary amine (RNH_2), an imine will form.

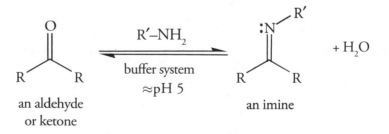

an aldehyde
or ketone

an imine

As in the acetal formation reaction, whatever R groups are originally attached to the carbonyl carbon stay attached in the product, and a molecule of water is liberated as a byproduct. A brief examination of the reaction mechanism will help illustrate these common features.

Mechanism

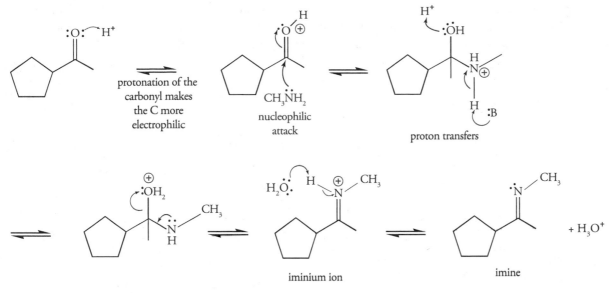

In the first step of this reaction, a lone pair of electrons on the carbonyl oxygen is protonated by the acidic medium. As in acetal formation, protonation of the carbonyl oxygen makes the carbonyl carbon more electrophilic and therefore more susceptible to nucleophilic attack. This time, the nucleophile is a primary amine, but attack by the nucleophilic nitrogen on the electrophilic carbon results in a similar tetrahedral intermediate. This intermediate is then deprotonated at the nitrogen and protonated at the oxygen, thereby converting a poor leaving group ($-OH$) into a good one ($-OH_2^+$). Next, the oxygen departs as a neutral water molecule, leaving behind a carbocation that is resonance-stabilized by the lone pair of electrons on nitrogen, reminiscent of the stabilization by the incoming oxygen during acetal formation. (*Note*: Only the more stable resonance form is shown in the mechanism above.) The similarities to acetal formation end here, as the final step of imine production is the deprotonation of the iminium ion to regenerate the acid catalyst.

Enamine Formation

While imines are derived from primary amines, if a secondary amine (R_2NH) is used under similar reaction conditions, the result is a functional group called an enamine. The overall reaction of a typical enamine synthesis is shown below. Note that this is another reversible reaction, and that enamines can be hydrolyzed to the carbonyl compound under aqueous acidic conditions.

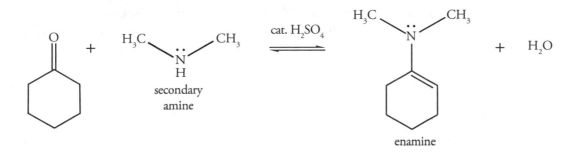

The mechanism of enamine formation is identical to imine formation until the final step. Since the in-coming amine is secondary rather than primary, the iminium ion cannot be deprotonated as in the imine mechanism. Instead, deprotonation of a hydrogen α to the double bond, now substantially more acidic on account of the positive charge on nitrogen, yields the enamine.

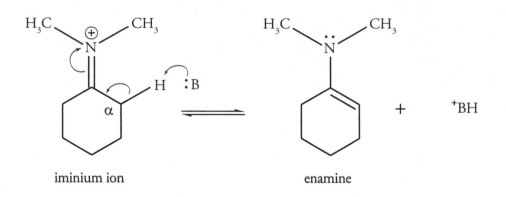

Enamines are a class of organic molecules resembling enols, in which the enol-oxygen of the aldehyde or ketone is replaced by a secondary amine. The chemistry of enamines is similar to enol chemistry in that it is largely governed by the resonance between the enamine and iminium structures. The partial double-bond character in the C—N bond, implied by the iminium resonance structure, results in the sp^2-hybridization of the enamine nitrogen and hindered rotation around the C—N bond (and the C—C$_\alpha$ bond in acyclic compounds).

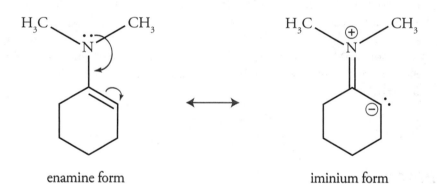

As the iminium resonance form above suggests, the α-carbon of the enamine is nucleophilic and will readily react with electrophiles. The increased donor ability of nitrogen, as compared to oxygen, results in enamines being more nucleophilic than neutral enols, but less nucleophilic than charged enolates (as we'll see shortly). As shown below, attack by the nucleophilic α-carbon on the polarized carbon of an alkyl halide results in the expulsion of the halide leaving group. This generates an iminium ion, which, as mentioned above, will reform the carbonyl under acidic, aqueous workup conditions.

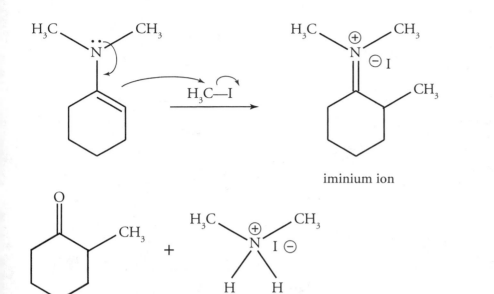

iminium ion

Example 6-5: Predict the major organic product of each of the following reactions:

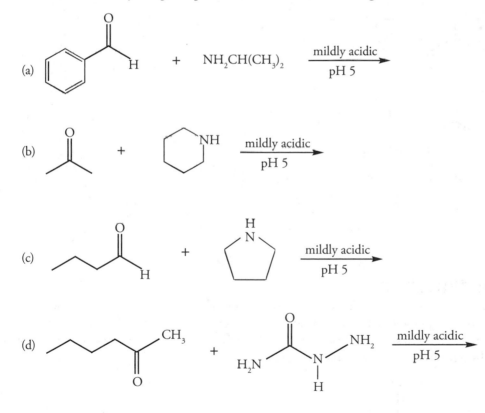

6.2

Solution:

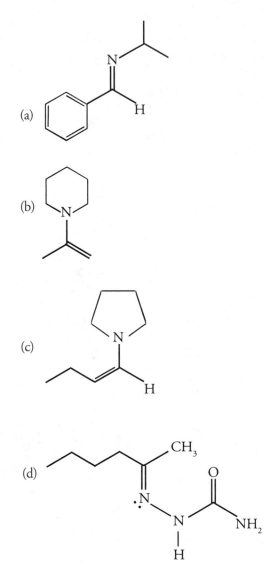

(a)

(b)

(c)

(d)

Aldol Condensation

A classic reaction in which the enolate anion of one carbonyl compound reacts with the carbonyl group of another carbonyl compound is called the aldol condensation. This reaction combines the two types of aldehyde/ketone reactivities: the acidity of the α-proton, and the electrophilicity of the carbonyl carbon, and forms a β-hydroxycarbonyl compound as the product.

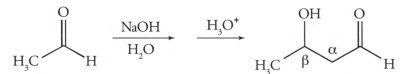

β–hydroxyaldehyde

As the mechanism below shows, in the first step of this reaction, a strong base removes an α-proton from the aldehyde or ketone, resulting in the formation of a resonance-stabilized enolate anion. (Remember, the enolate anion is nucleophilic and usually reacts at the carbon atom that was deprotonated.) Next, the α-carbon of the enolate anion attacks the carbonyl carbon of another aldehyde molecule, thereby generating an alkoxide ion that is subsequently protonated by a molecule of water. This results in the formation of a general class of molecules referred to as β-hydroxy carbonyl compounds.

The Mechanism

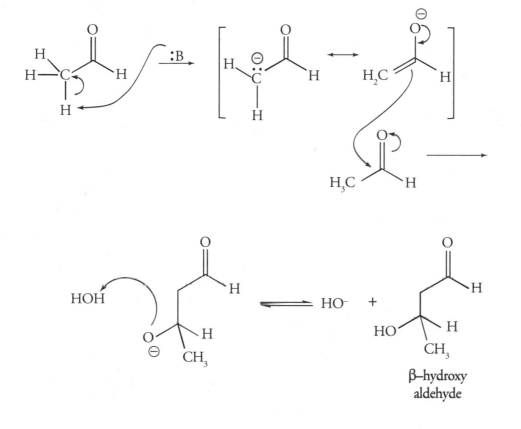

β–hydroxy
aldehyde

There are three important points to note about this reaction. First, it requires a strong base (typically hydroxide, OH⁻ or an alkoxide ion RO⁻) to remove an α-proton adjacent to the carbonyl group. Second, one of the aldehydes or ketones must act as a source for the enolate ions while the other aldehyde or ketone will come under nucleophilic attack by the enolate carbanion. Third, the aldol condensation does not require the two carbonyl groups that participate in the reaction to be the same. When they are different, it is called a **crossed aldol condensation** reaction. In order to avoid obtaining a complex mixture of products in a crossed aldol condensation, it is often the case that one of the carbonyl compounds is chosen such that it does not have any acidic α-protons, and therefore *cannot* act as the nucleophile (enolate ion), it *must* be the electrophile.

Kinetic vs. Thermodynamic Control of the Aldol Reaction

When asymmetric ketones with more than one set of α-protons are treated with base, two different eno-lates are possible. When these ketones are used to perform aldol reactions, different products are formed depending on which enolate is used. Regiochemical control of such a reaction can be achieved through the choice of base and the reaction conditions, as depicted below.

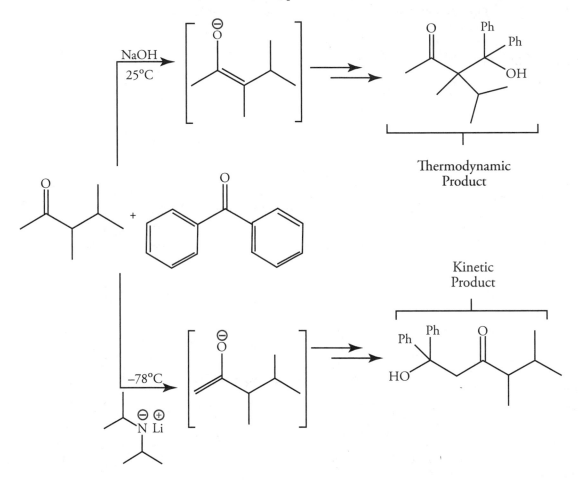

The upper-pathway, run at room temperature with an unencumbered base, is said to be under *thermodynamic* control. In general, double bonds with more carbon-substituents (fewer vinyl-hydrogens) are more thermodynamically stable than less-substituted alkenes. In the absence of other constraints, the enolate formed by removing protons from the more sterically crowded α-carbon will be favored.

Formation of the less-substituted enolate (the lower-pathway) may be achieved by denying the base access to the more sterically hindered α-carbon. Two ways to do this include using a bulky base that cannot fit into the area required to remove the sterically-shielded proton (in this case, lithium diisopropyl amide, or LDA), or by doing the reaction at very low temperature. At a reduced temperature, there is not enough energy to overcome the activation barrier associated with the base approaching the more crowded α-carbon. Through use of these constraints, the base will deprotonate the less hindered, more kinetically accessible α-carbon. These reactions are said to be under **kinetic control**.

Retro-Aldol Reaction and Dehydration

Though stabilized by an intramolecular hydrogen bond between the hydroxyl and carbonyl groups, and hence generally thermodynamically stable at moderate temperatures and pH levels, β-hydroxy aldehydes and ketones are not immune to further transformations. When treated with strong bases, deprotonation of the free hydroxyl group may induce the reverse of the initial aldol condensation in a reaction known as a retro-aldol reaction. It is useful to note that the constitutive pieces of any β-hydroxy aldehyde or ketone synthesized via an aldol reaction may be determined by working through the mechanism of the retro-aldol.

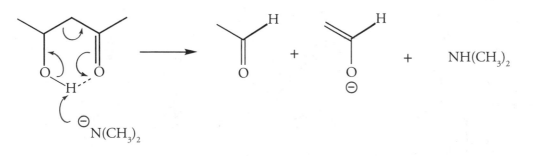

If the β-hydroxyaldehyde or ketone products are heated, they will undergo an elimination reaction (dehydration) to form an α,β-**unsaturated carbonyl compound**. Notice that the newly formed carbon-carbon π bond is in conjugation with the carbonyl group; this stabilizes the molecule.

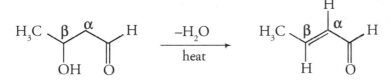

β-hydroxy carbonyl   α,β-unsaturated carbonyl compound
(some Z compound will also form)

6.2

Example 6-6: Predict the condensation products of each of the following reactions. Show both the β-hydroxy carbonyl product and the elimination product.

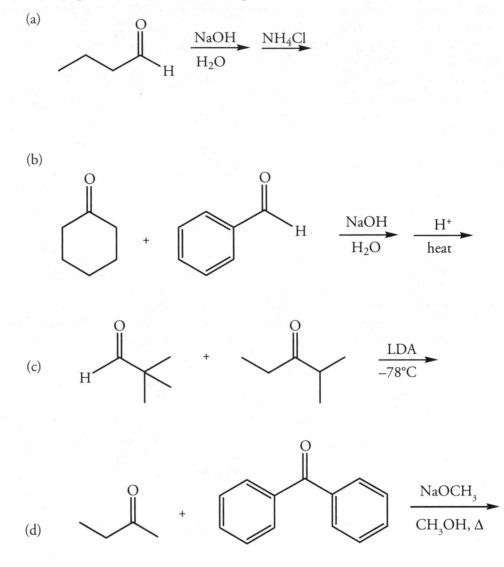

(a)

(b)

(c)

(d)

CARBONYL CHEMISTRY

Solution:

(a)

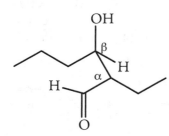 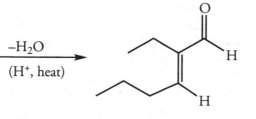

$$-H_2O$$
$$(H^+, \text{heat})$$

(b)

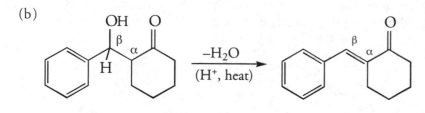

$$-H_2O$$
$$(H^+, \text{heat})$$

(c)

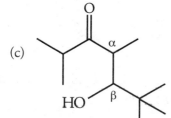 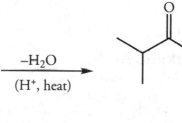

$$-H_2O$$
$$(H^+, \text{heat})$$

(d)

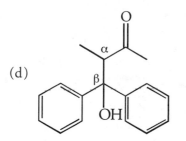 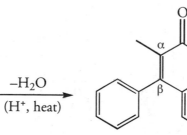 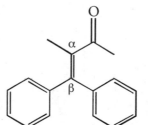

$$-H_2O$$
$$(H^+, \text{heat})$$

6.3 CARBOXYLIC ACIDS

Carboxylic acids are of fundamental importance in many biological systems. Fatty acids, for example, are long chain carboxylic acids that play important roles in both cellular structure and metabolism (as we'll see in Section 7.4). In the following sections, we'll explore the basic physical properties and common chemical reactions of carboxylic acids and their derivatives.

Hydrogen Bonding

Carboxylic acids form strong hydrogen bonds because the carboxylate group contains both a hydrogen bond donor and a hydrogen bond acceptor. This can be seen in the intermolecular hydrogen bonding of acetic acid. Notice that the acidic proton is the hydrogen bond donor and a lone pair of electrons on the carbonyl oxygen is the hydrogen bond acceptor. For this reason, carboxylic acids can form stable hydrogen bonded dimers, giving them high melting and boiling points.

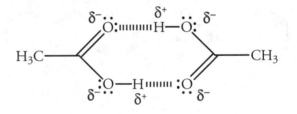

Reduction of Carboxylic Acids

Earlier in the chapter we discussed the use of boron and aluminum hydrides in the reduction of ketones and aldehydes to their respective alcohols. Carboxylic acids can similarly be reduced to primary alcohols, with one important difference: $LiAlH_4$ is effective, but $NaBH_4$ is not.

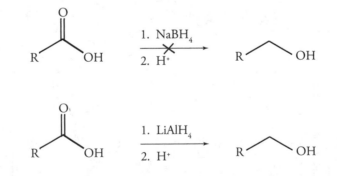

As aluminum is slightly more electropositive than boron, the Al—H bond is more highly polarized, more reductive, and ultimately capable of performing these more challenging reductions.

Decarboxylation Reactions of β-Keto Acids

Carboxylic acids that have carbonyl groups β to the carboxylate are unstable because they are subject to decarboxylation. The reaction proceeds through a cyclic transition state and results in the loss of carbon dioxide from the β-keto acid.

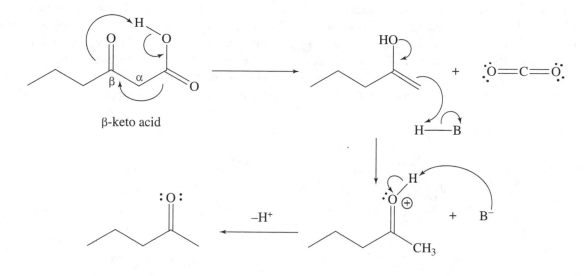

β-keto acid

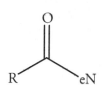

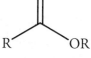

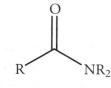

6.4 CARBOXYLIC ACID DERIVATIVES

Carboxylic acid derivatives include acid chlorides, acid anhydrides, esters, and amides. The general chemical structures for these acid derivatives are:

(eN = electronegative group)

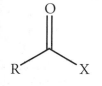

X = halogen
acid halide

acid
anhydride

ester

amide

As you might expect, the derivatives of carboxylic acids react similarly to aldehydes because they are also electrophilic at the carbonyl carbon atom. However, unlike reactions with aldehydes and ketones, nucleophilic additions to carboxylic acid derivatives are usually followed by elimination. (Note that additions and eliminations are opposites—while you can recognize an addition reaction because a π bond is broken and replaced by two new σ bonds, eliminations are the reverse. A new π bond is formed while two σ bonds break.) This is because the tetrahedral intermediate formed upon attack of the nucleophile on the carbonyl carbon has both a negatively charged oxygen atom (the former carbonyl oxygen), and a good leaving group (the eN-group of the carboxylic acid derivative). This elimination by the electrons on the oxygen atom regenerates the carbonyl, thereby displacing the leaving group (eN⁻). This is called a **nucleophilic addition-elimination reaction,** and is sometimes referred to as an acyl substitution.

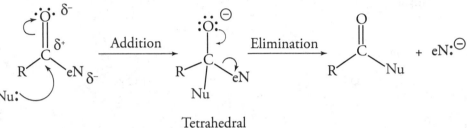

| Acid derivative | Tetrahedral intermediate | New acid derivative |

Esterification Reactions

An **esterification reaction** occurs when a carboxylic acid reacts with an alcohol in the presence of a catalytic amount of acid.

Esterification

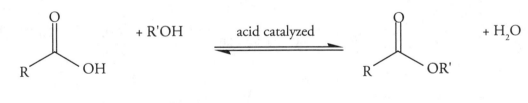

a carboxylic acid   an alcohol   an ester

The following mechanism shows that protonation of the carbonyl oxygen makes the carbonyl carbon more electrophilic, and nucleophilic attack by the oxygen of the alcohol results in a tetrahedral intermediate that is neutralized by deprotonation. An –OH group of the tetrahedral intermediate is then protonated, converting a poor leaving group (–OH) into a good one ($-OH_2^+$). As a result, a water molecule departs, leaving behind the protonated form of the ester. Deprotonation of the carbonyl oxygen yields the ester product and regenerates the acid catalyst.

The Acid-Catalyzed Mechanism

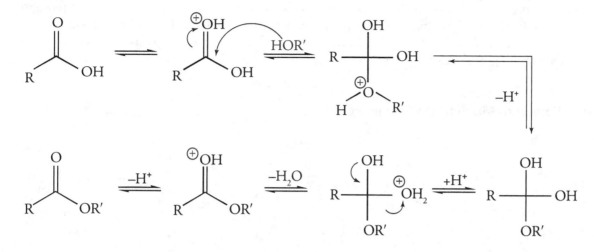

Acidic and Basic Hydrolysis of Esters

Let's now examine both the acidic and basic hydrolysis of the ester *methyl benzoate* to form the carboxylic acid and alcohol. First, we look at the acid-catalyzed reaction:

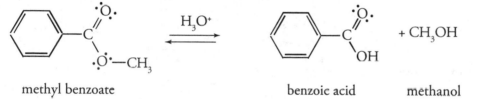

| methyl benzoate | benzoic acid | methanol |

In the first step of this reaction, the carbonyl oxygen is protonated. As before, the protonation of the carbonyl oxygen makes the carbon more electrophilic. Nucleophilic attack by a water molecule, followed by deprotonation, leads to the formation of a tetrahedral intermediate. *In any nucleophilic addition-elimination reaction of an acid derivative, there will always be a tetrahedral intermediate.*

Acid-Catalyzed Ester Hydrolysis Mechanism

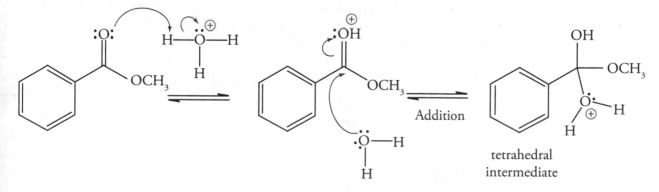

Next, the leaving group of the tetrahedral intermediate is protonated under the acidic reaction conditions. Notice that protonation of the hydroxyl oxygens can also occur. This leads to the reverse reaction. Protonation of the leaving group converts a poor leaving group (RO⁻, an alkoxide ion) into a good one (ROH, a neutral alcohol molecule). The alcohol leaves and yields a protonated acid that only has to undergo a deprotonation to give the carboxylic acid product.

Acid-Catalyzed Mechanism, Continued

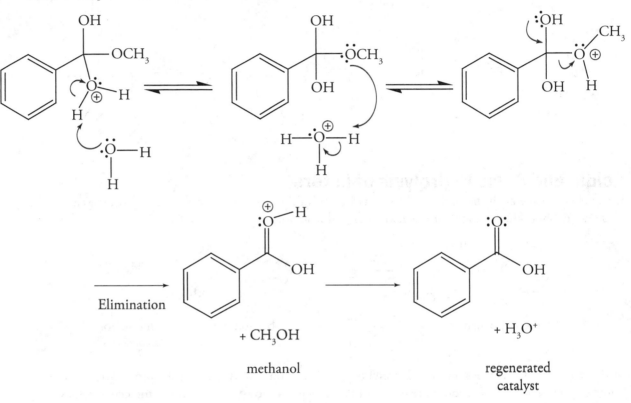

Elimination

+ CH₃OH

methanol

+ H₃O⁺

regenerated
catalyst

Transesterification

Not only can esters be hydrolyzed to carboxylic acids, but treatment of esters with alcohols, generally with acid catalysis, results in a process known as transesterification. Following an equivalent mechanism as shown above for hydrolysis, the nucleophilic attack by an alcohol on the electrophilic carbonyl-carbon of the ester results in the replacement of the original –OR (below depicted as EtO–) with the incoming alcohol (depicted below as isobutanol).

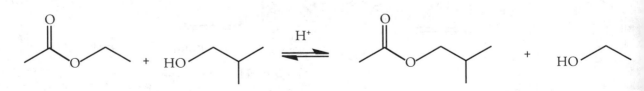

Like the esterification/hydrolysis reactions, the two esters exist in equilibrium, but there are a number of ways to favor the formation of the desired ester. One way is to employ conditions that remove by-products of the reaction from solution. For example, since ethanol is more volatile than isobutanol, mildly heating the reaction on the previous page will drive ethanol into the vapor phase and push the reaction to the right via Le Châtelier's principle. Similarly, using a large excess of the alcohol constituting the desired –OR in the product serves to shift the equilibrium in the desired direction. Such conditions are indicated as in the equation below.

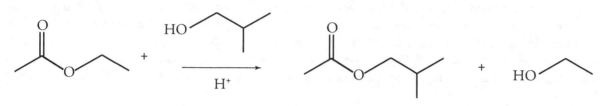

Placing isobutanol above or below the arrow denotes that it is used as the solvent, and is therefore in great excess. As a result, the equilibrium is essentially halted and the reaction is driven completely to the right. The reverse reaction is, of course, still possible if the isobutanol solvent is removed and replaced with ethanol.

Base-Mediated Ester Hydrolysis Mechanism

We now consider the corresponding *base*-mediated hydrolysis of methyl benzoate. In the first step of the reaction, the strongly nucleophilic hydroxide ion directly attacks the electrophilic carbonyl carbon. The nucleophilic attack results in the formation of a tetrahedral intermediate.

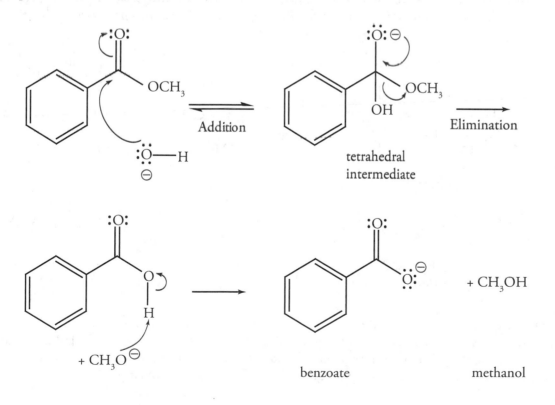

The tetrahedral intermediate then undergoes an elimination reaction, reforming the carbonyl when a pair of electrons on the negatively charged oxygen regenerates the carbon-oxygen π bond. This eliminates the alkoxide ion as a leaving group. However, since the reaction is carried out under basic conditions and the alkoxide ion is a strong enough base to deprotonate the newly formed carboxylic acid, the final step of the mechanism is the acid-base reaction shown on the previous page. In order to recover the carboxylic acid from this process, the reaction must have a final aqueous acidic workup.

In summary, these two reactions, the acid-catalyzed hydrolysis of an ester and the base-mediated hydrolysis of an ester, display the most common reactivities of all of the carboxylic acid derivatives. Both of these reactions give the same products, but by different mechanisms. Most importantly, both of the mechanisms proceed through nucleophilic addition and elimination steps. A good understanding of these two reaction mechanisms leads to a solid understanding of all of the reactions of carboxylic acids and their derivatives.

Saponification: An Example of a Base-Mediated Ester Hydrolysis Reaction

The hydrolysis of fats and glycerides is a chemical reaction that has been practiced for many centuries in the process of making soap. Typically, large vats of animal fat are treated with lye (NaOH or KOH) and stirred over a roaring fire. This bubbling cauldron liberates free fatty acids from the animal fat, which then can be utilized as soap.

Upon inspection, it is clear that this ancient method is simply the basic hydrolysis of a triacylglyceride to yield a molecule of glycerol and three fatty acids. This is the reaction mechanism we just reviewed.

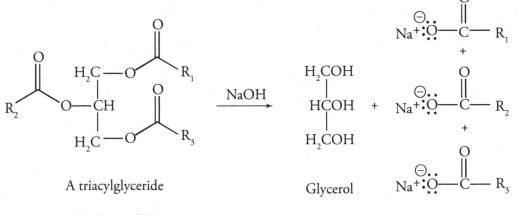

A triacylglyceride

(R_1, R_2, and R_3 can be the same or different.)

Glycerol

Fatty acids

The three electrophilic carbonyl carbons of the triacylglyceride sequentially undergo nucleophilic attack by hydroxide ions to produce an oxy-anion tetrahedral intermediate. Then the tetrahedral intermediate eliminates the —OR portion of the ester as an alkoxide ion which is then protonated to form the alcohol. This happens three times to ultimately yield glycerol and three molecules of fatty acid.

Fatty acids are **amphipathic** molecules, because they contain a negatively charged carboxylate group that is hydrophilic and a long hydrocarbon tail that's hydrophobic. As a result, these amphipathic fatty acid molecules form micelles in water in which the hydrophobic tails associate with one another to exclude water, while the charged carboxylate groups are localized on the exterior of the micelles. Greases and fats are adsorbed by the fatty portion of these micelles and the whole micelle is "washed" away by water. This is the physical basis of soap. We will discuss this further in Chapter 7.

Synthesis of the Carboxylic Acid Derivatives

Now that we understand how the electronic structure of the carboxylic acid derivatives relates to their reactivity, the synthesis of carboxylic acid derivatives should be straightforward. For the most part, we shall only be concerned with the interconversion of one derivative to another.

Acid Halides

Carboxylic acid halides are made from the corresponding carboxylic acid and either $SOCl_2$ or PX_3 (X = Cl, Br).

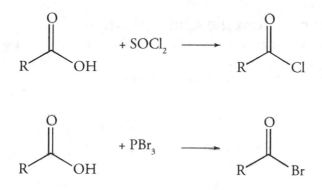

Acid Anhydrides

As their name implies, anhydrides (meaning "without water") can be prepared by the condensation of two carboxylic acids with the loss of water.

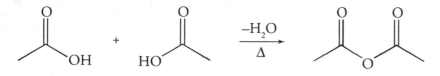

Acid anhydrides are also prepared from addition of the corresponding carboxylic acid (or carboxylate ion) to the corresponding acid halide.

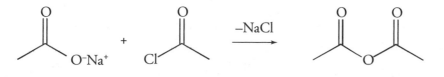

6.4

Esters

Esters are most easily synthesized from the corresponding carboxylic acid and an alcohol, as we saw earlier. This reaction is referred to as **esterification**. Esters can also be prepared from an acid halide, an anhydride, or another ester and a corresponding alcohol.

Amides

Amides can be prepared from the corresponding acid halide, anhydride, or ester with the desired amine. They *cannot* be prepared from the carboxylic acid directly. This is because amines are very basic, and carboxylic acids are very acidic; an acid-base reaction occurs much faster than the desired addition-elimination reaction.

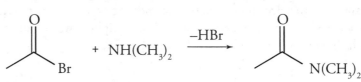

Carboxylic acids can be prepared from *any* of the derivatives merely by heating the derivative in acidic aqueous solutions.

Relative Reactivity of Carboxylic Acid Derivatives

Now that we are familiar with the general reactivity of carboxylic acid derivatives, we will examine how chemical *structure* affects the *relative* chemical reactivity of common acid derivatives. The order of reactivity in nucleophilic addition-elimination reactions for acid derivatives is:

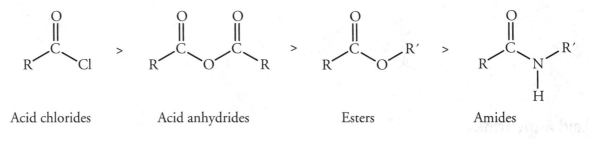

| Acid chlorides | Acid anhydrides | Esters | Amides |

If we examine the leaving groups of these acid derivatives, it is clear that the reactivity of acid derivatives in nucleophilic addition-elimination reactions decreases with increasing basicity of the leaving group.

Acid Derivative Reactivity

Acid Derivative	*Leaving Group*	
 acid chloride	Cl⊖	Chloride anion is a very good leaving group. It is a very weak base since it is the conjugate base of the strong acid HCl ($pK_a = -7$).
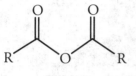 acid anhydride		This is a fairly good leaving group. It is the conjugate base of the weakly acidic carboxylic acid ($pK_a = 4–5$).
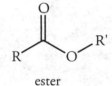 ester	⊖:Ö—R	An alkoxide ion is a rather poor leaving group. It is moderately basic since it is the conjugate base of alcohol, which is a fairly weak acid ($pK_a = 15–19$).
amide	⊖:N̈—R' H	This is a horrible leaving group. It is strongly basic since it is the conjugate base of an amine, which is a terrible acid ($pK_a = 35–40$).

While acid chlorides and anhydrides are readily hydrolyzed in water, esters and amides are much more stable. Esters require either acidic or basic conditions and elevated temperatures in order to effect hydrolysis, and amides are generally only hydrolyzed under acidic conditions, high temperatures, and long reaction times.

Chapter 6 Summary

- The C=O bond is very polarized due to the high electronegativity of oxygen, resulting in the carbon of the carbonyl group being electrophilic.

- Protons α to a carbonyl are acidic and can be removed by a strong base to yield a nucleophilic carbanion, or enolate.

- Keto-enol tautomerism is the rapid equilibration of the more stable keto form of a carbonyl and the less stable enol form where the α-proton shifts to the carbonyl oxygen.

- Nucleophilic additions involve the attack of a nucleophile on the carbon of an aldehyde or ketone; these reactions break one π bond to form two σ bonds.

- Hydride reduction, a type of nucleophilic addition, can convert ketones or aldehydes into alcohols; alcohols can be converted back to carbonyl compounds using oxidizing agents.

- An aldol condensation is a C—C bond forming reaction where the carbonyl carbon of one molecule is the electrophile, while the α-carbon of another carbonyl compound is the nucleophile.

- The formation of a specific enolate from an asymmetrical ketone can be controlled by carefully manipulating reaction conditions. The less substituted (kinetic) enolate is formed at low temperatures with bulky bases, while the more substituted (thermodynamic) enolate is formed at higher temperatures with small bases.

- The reactivity of carboxylic acid derivatives decreases as follows: acid halide > acid anhydride > ester > amide.

- Nucleophilic addition to the carbonyl carbon in a carboxylic acid derivative is usually followed by elimination due to the presence of a good electronegative leaving group.

CHAPTER 6 FREESTANDING PRACTICE QUESTIONS

1. Rank the protons from least acidic to most acidic.

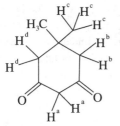

A) $H^a < H^b = H^d < H^c$
B) $H^c < H^d < H^b < H^a$
C) $H^c < H^b = H^d < H^a$
D) $H^c < H^b < H^d < H^a$

2. Predict a possible product of the following reaction:

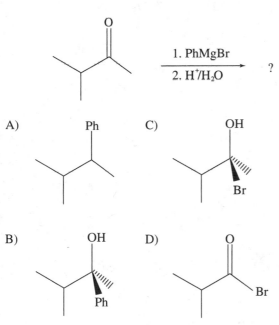

1. PhMgBr
2. H^+/H_2O

?

A) Ph

C) OH
Br

B) OH
Ph

D) O
Br

3. The enol and keto tautomers of 3-pentanone (shown below) are best described as:

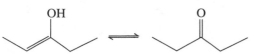

A) resonance structures.
B) geometric isomers.
C) constitutional isomers.
D) diastereomers.

4. Which of the following carbonyl compounds cannot undergo a self aldol condensation?

A) 2,2,4,4-tetramethylpentan-3-one
B) 1,2,2-triphenylethanone
C) 3,3-dimethylbutan-2-one
D) pentan-2-one

5. Which of the following would increase the rate of the reaction shown below?

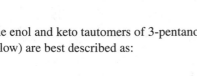

EtOH

I. Addition of acid
II. Addition of base
III. Increased concentration of EtOH

A) I only
B) I and II only
C) I and III only
D) I, II, and III

CHAPTER 6 PRACTICE PASSAGE

The *Robinson annulation* reaction is a widely used, multi-step process for generating cyclic α,β-unsaturated ketones. The first step (known as a *Michael reaction*) involves conjugate addition of an enol or enolate to an α,β-unsaturated carbonyl (Molecule 1). The reaction then proceeds with ring closure and loss of water (cyclodehydration) to give a cyclic α,β-unsaturated ketone (Molecule 8).

Scientists have found a way to catalyze the Robinson annulation by using artificial enzymes made from antibodies (Zhong, *et. al., J. Am. Chem. Soc.* 1997, *119*, 8131). As shown in Figure 1, these catalytic antibodies speed up the reaction by using a lysine side chain to form an imine with Molecule 3. The imine more readily undergoes tautomerization and cyclodehydration to give Molecule 7, which is easily hydrolyzed to Molecule 8. An important result is that Molecule 8 is produced as a single enantiomer.

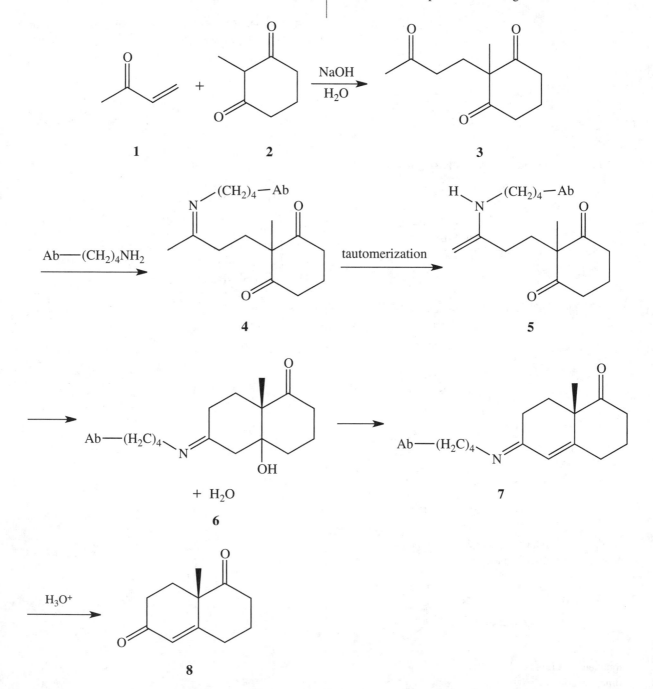

Figure 1 Enzymatic catalysis of Robinson annulation

1. In the first step shown in Figure 1, which of the following acts as the nucleophile?

A) Enol of Molecule 1
B) Enolate of Molecule 1
C) Enol of Molecule 2
D) Enolate of Molecule 2

2. The antibody described in the passage catalyzes an enantioselective Robinson annulation reaction. What is the stereochemistry of the single enantiomer that is produced?

A) (E)-(R)
B) (E)-(S)
C) (Z)-(R)
D) (Z)-(S)

3. The reaction of Molecule 3 with the lysine side chain of the catalytic antibody can best be described as what type of reaction?

A) Hydrolysis
B) Alkylation
C) Addition–elimination
D) Esterification

4. If the first step in Figure 1 was carried out in NaOD/D$_2$O, which of the following molecules would NOT be produced?

A)

B)

C)

D)

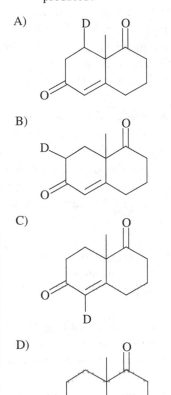

5. An aldol condensation between which two compounds could be used to generate Molecule 1?

A)

B)

C)

D)

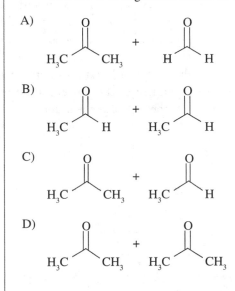

SOLUTIONS TO CHAPTER 6 FREESTANDING PRACTICE QUESTIONS

1. **C**   Because H^a is bound to a carbon that is adjacent to two carbonyl groups, it is the easiest proton for a base to abstract since the conjugate base has the most resonance structures. Therefore, you can eliminate choice A. Because this molecule has a mirror plane, H^b and H^d are equivalent, so you can eliminate choices B and D, which leaves choice C as the correct choice. H^c is on a carbon that is not adjacent to any electron withdrawing groups or pi electrons, so it is the least acidic.

2. **B**   This is an addition reaction involving a ketone and a Grignard reagent (RMgX). The R-group in the Grignard reagent, in this case the phenyl, adds on to the carbonyl carbon, and the acid workup step is used to protonate the carbonyl oxygen into an alcohol. This gives the product shown in choice B. Choice A can be eliminated as ketones cannot undergo substitution reactions with Grignard reagents due to lack of an appropriate leaving group. Choices C and D can be eliminated since the halogen is not the nucleophilic atom in a Grignard reagent.

3. **C**   Tautomers do not have the same connectivity of atoms; they are constitutional isomers which are in equilibrium with one another. Choices A, B, and D all have the same connectivity of atoms.

4. **A**   A self aldol condensation occurs between two molecules of the same compound. In order for an aldol condensation to occur, at least one of the carbonyl compounds must be able to form an enolate through deprotonation of an α-carbon. Since 2,2,4,4-tetramethylpentan-3-one contains no α-hydrogens, it cannot form an enolate, and therefore cannot undergo a self-condensation reaction. All of the other molecules listed have at least one α-hydrogen, and therefore can undergo self-condensation reactions.

5. **A**   Although hemiacetal formation is catalyzed by both acid and base, conversion of the hemiacetal to the acetal requires a catalytic amount of acid to protonate the hemiacetal OH group so it can leave as water. The presence of base would prevent this from occurring, and slow acetal formation. Therefore, choices B and D can be eliminated, and Item I is true; it catalyzes both hemiacetal and acetal formation. Although hemiacetal formation occurs through nucleophilic addition, a bimolecular mechanism that involves both the carbonyl compound and the nucleophile (in this case, EtOH), the rate limiting step of this reaction is the conversion of the hemiacetal to the acetal. This conversion requires formation of a high-energy carbocation intermediate. Therefore, the kinetics of the rate limiting step are independent of the concentration of EtOH, and increasing its concentration would not increase the rate of the reaction.

SOLUTIONS TO CHAPTER 6 PRACTICE PASSAGE

1. **D** As the passage states, the first step of the reaction involves the conjugate addition of an enol or enolate to an α,β-unsaturated carbonyl. Since Molecule 1 is the α,β-unsaturated carbonyl (the electrophile), Molecule 2 must act as the nucleophilic enol or enolate. Given the basic conditions, the enolate of Molecule 2 will be formed.

2. **D** The alkene product (Molecule 8) has both highest-priority groups on the same side of the double bond, giving it (*Z*) stereochemistry so eliminate answer choices A and B. To assign (*R*) or (*S*) configuration to the single stereocenter, we must first assign priority to its substituents according to the Cahn-Ingold-Prelog Rules for assigning stereochemistry (see below).

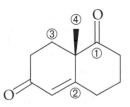

Now, looking down the bond from the stereocenter to the lowest-priority group (from below the plane of the page), the substituents progress from highest to lowest priority in a counterclockwise direction, giving this stereocenter the (*S*) configuration.

3. **C** Formation of the imine from Molecule 3 begins with addition of the nucleophilic lysine nitrogen atom to the electrophilic carbonyl group. Water is then eliminated to complete formation of the imine.

4. **A** In the presence of a base, enolates can be reversibly formed, resulting in deuterium labeling at the α-carbons in the first step of the reaction. Thus, the α-carbons labeled a (choice C), b (choice B), c, d (choice D), and e, shown below, may all be deuterated:

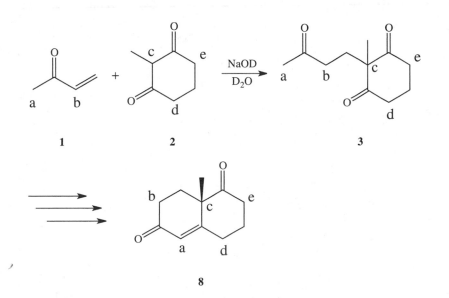

Since the position labeled in choice A is not an α-carbon and cannot be deprotonated, it will not be deuterated.

5. **A** An aldol condensation between an enol and ketone or aldehyde yields an α,β-unsaturated carbonyl compound. The alkene marks the newly-formed bond between the two molecules. Therefore, using retrosynthetic analysis of Molecule 1, we see that it may be formed from acetone and formaldehyde (choice A).

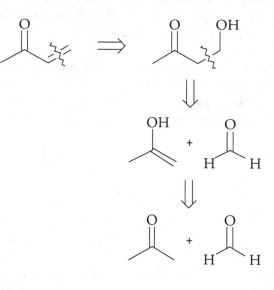

Chapter 7
Biologically Important
Molecules

INTRODUCTION

As you begin reading and working through this chapter of the text, you will notice that it is a little different than the other chapters. Up to now, this book has presented you with lots of information, then offered you practice questions and passages to help you test yourself. But this book's real purpose is not to just stuff you with detail—it is to make you think. Thus, this chapter is written in a style intended to do just that.

This chapter offers you *grillage*; that is, it puts you "on the grill" by asking you questions on the material you're reading and studying. In other words, the approach is Socratic. The grillage takes the form of questions between paragraphs, but also rears its head as queries that interrupt the flow of text. Some of the questions test factual knowledge that has already been presented. Others ask you to speculate, based on new information. Others force you to integrate factual knowledge and speculation. The idea is to wake you up and remind you that you're not supposed to be memorizing, but rather thinking about the information flowing past your eyes, speculating about it, integrating it with what you know, what you'd like to know, and what you'd like to do with all that knowledge (help sick people).

It is crucial that you take advantage of the grillage. How? When the book asks you a question, you'll usually find the answer in a footnote on the same page. DON'T READ THE FOOTNOTE UNTIL YOU'VE ANSWERED THE QUESTION! Some of the answers are as simple as "C" or "No," and others are complex conceptual explanations. In any case, take the time to formulate a thorough answer before you go to the footnote. If you think you're too rushed to "waste" time doing this, we've got news for you: you are studying the wrong way. The real waste of time is doing nothing but memorizing details. The profitable time is spent pondering concepts, as you'll do on the day of the MCAT. Though you shouldn't read the footnotes too soon, do be sure to read them, as sometimes they contain important information or vocabulary not given in the main body of the text.

7.1 AMINO ACIDS

Proteins are biological macromolecules that act as enzymes, hormones, receptors, antibodies, and support structures inside and outside cells. Proteins are composed of twenty different amino acids linked together in polymers. The composition and sequence of amino acids in the polypeptide chain is what makes each protein unique and enables it to fulfill its special role in the cell. In this section of Chapter 7, we will start with amino acids, the building blocks of proteins, and work our way up to three-dimensional protein structure and function.

Amino Acid Structure and Nomenclature

Understanding the structure of amino acids is key to understanding both their chemistry and the chemistry of proteins. The generic formula for all twenty amino acids is shown below.

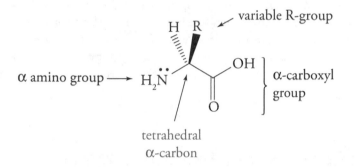

Generic Amino Acid Structure

All twenty amino acids share the same nitrogen-carbon-carbon backbone. The unique feature of each amino acid is its **side chain** (variable R-group), which gives it the physical and chemical properties that distinguish it from the other nineteen. Note that the α-carbon of each of the twenty amino acids is a stereocenter (has four different groups), except in the case of glycine, whose α-carbon is bonded to two hydrogen atoms. This means that all of the amino acids are chiral except for glycine.

L- and D-Amino Acids

Chemists often draw chiral molecules in their **Fischer projection** to illustrate stereochemistry. Let's review how Fischer projections denote the absolute stereochemistry of molecules. The conformation of a molecule that is shown in a Fischer projection happens to be the least stable, fully eclipsed form of the molecule. In Fischer projections the most oxidized carbon is at the top, and the structure is extended vertically until the final carbon atom is reached. This leaves the substituents on each carbon atom to occupy the horizontal positions of each carbon atom in the chain. This is illustrated on the next page.

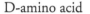

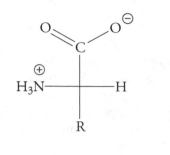

L-amino acid

D-amino acid

In the Fischer projection, it's understood that all horizontal lines are projecting from the plane of the page toward the viewer, and all vertical lines are projecting into the plane of the page, away from the viewer.

All animal amino acids are of the L-configuration, with the amino group drawn on the Left in Fischer nota-tion. Some **D**-amino acids, with the amino group on the right, occur in a few specialized structures, such as bacterial cell walls. The L and D classification system can be a source of great confusion. For the MCAT, it is most important to remember that *all animal amino acids have the L configuration and that all naturally occurring carbohydrates have the D configuration.* (Carbohydrates are discussed in a later section of this chapter.) For completeness, though, we'll take the time to discuss the meaning of D and L now.

Assigning the Configuration to a Chiral Center

L- and D-amino acids and L- and D-carbohydrates are **enantiomeric stereoisomers**. The simplest (small-est) carbohydrate has only three carbons and only one chiral center. It is called **glyceraldehyde**. Since it has one chiral center, this molecule can exist in one of two enantiomeric forms, (+)-glyceraldehyde and (–)-glyceraldehyde. In reactions occurring in living organisms, CHOH groups are added to carbon #1 of glyceraldehyde to form larger carbohydrate molecules with more than one chiral center. In this synthetic process the configuration at the original glyceraldehyde chiral carbon (#2) is not changed. So, if you start with (–)-glyceraldehyde and build a longer carbohydrate chain, that carbohydrate chain will have a pen-ultimate (second-to-last) carbon atom with the same configuration as (–)-glyceraldehyde. So why not just call the new, larger carbohydrate "(–)"? You cannot refer to the new carbohydrate as (–) because you have added several new chiral centers, and now if you put the new molecule in solution and measure its optical rotation with a polarimeter, the optical activity may in fact be (+). What is needed is a way to name a car-bohydrate that would specify that it had been built up from (–)- or (+)-glyceraldehyde without worrying about its actual optical activity.

L-(–)-Glyceraldehyde

D-(+)-Glyceraldehyde

The solution is to nickname (–)-glyceraldehyde as "L-glyceraldehyde," and to likewise refer to (+)-glyceraldehyde as "D-glyceraldehyde." Now we can refer to all carbohydrates built up from (–)-glyceraldehyde as "L" carbohydrates, without specifying whether they rotate plane-polarized light to the left (–) or to the right (+). All we have to do is look at the last chiral carbon in the chain and decide whether it looks like C2 from L- or D-glyceraldehyde.

Once again, the important thing to remember is that *all animal amino acids are derived from L-glyceraldehyde* (because they share the same basic structure at the penultimate carbon). Hence, they all have the L configuration. *Animal carbohydrates are chemically derived from D-glyceraldehyde*, and are thus all D.

As we discussed in Chapter 3, there is another classification system, in which chiral centers are denoted either *R* or *S*. This system describes the *absolute configuration* of the chiral center; it refers to the actual three-dimensional arrangement of groups, as in a model or drawing; it says nothing about what the molecule will do to plane-polarized light.

In summary, you can see that three classification systems are used to organize amino acids and carbohydrates:

1. (+) and (–) describe optical activity, and mean the same thing as *d* and *l*, respectively;
2. *R* and *S* describe actual structure or absolute configuration; and
3. D and L tell us the basic precursor of a molecule (D- or L-glyceraldehyde).

You can also see that the three different classification systems don't describe each other in any way. A molecule that has the *R* configuration of its only stereocenter might rotate plane-polarized light *either* clockwise *or* counterclockwise, and hence be *either* (+) *or* (–). And a molecule that is experimentally determined to be (+) might be either D or L. However, two of the three classification systems go together for certain molecules. All D-sugars have the *R* configuration at the penultimate carbon atom because they are all derived from D-glyceraldehyde. Similarly, all L-sugars have the *S* configuration at the penultimate carbon atom. This is true only because carbohydrates are named according to the configuration of the last chiral center in the chain (which, remember, is synthetically derived from glyceraldehyde). By the same rationale, all L-amino acids are *S*, and all D-amino acids are *R*. (Note that the only exception is for cysteine, because the R group (CH_2SH) of this amino acid has a higher priority than the COOH group.)

1) You crash-land on Mars without any food but notice that Mars is loaded with edible-looking plants. Martian life has evolved with all L-carbohydrates. Can you metabolize carbohydrates from Mars?[1]

---

[1] No. Enzyme activity depends on three-dimensional shape, and all animal digestive enzymes have active sites specific for substrate carbohydrates with the D configuration.

Classification of Amino Acids

Each of the twenty amino acids is unique because of its side chain, but many of them are similar in their chemical properties. You should be familiar with the side chains, and it is important to understand the chemical properties that characterize them, such as their varying *shape, ability to hydrogen bond, and ability to act as acids or bases (which determines their charge at physiological pH).*

As you study the 20 amino acids, do so by organizing them into four broad categories: ACIDIC, BASIC, NONPOLAR, and POLAR amino acids. Each amino acid has a three-letter abbreviation and a one-letter abbreviation, which are both important to know for the MCAT. This may seem like a lot of trivia to keep track of, but if you prioritize memorizing the codes of the acidic and basic amino acids, you are likely to be able to answer the vast majority of amino acid-related MCAT questions.

Acidic Amino Acids

Aspartic acid and glutamic acid are the only amino acids with carboxylic acid functional groups ($pK_a \approx 4$) in their side chains, thereby making the side chains acidic. Thus, there are three functional groups in these amino acids that may act as acids—the two backbone groups and the R-group. You may hear the terms aspart*ate* and glutam*ate*—these simply refer to the anionic (deprotonated) form of each molecule, which is how these amino acids are observed at physiological pH.

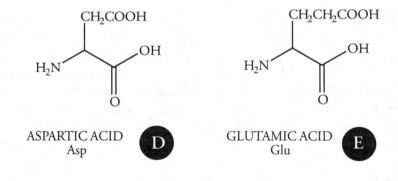

Basic Amino Acids

Lysine, arginine, and histidine have basic R-group side chains. The pK_a values for the side chains in these amino acids are 10 for Lys, 12 for Arg, and 6.5 for His. Both Lys and Arg are cationic (protonated) at physiological pH, but histidine is unique in having a side chain with a pK_a close to physiological pH. At pH 7.4, histidine may be either protonated or deprotonated—we put it in the basic category, but it often acts as an acid, too. This makes it a readily available proton acceptor or donor, explaining its prevalence at protein active sites. A mnemonic is "His goes both ways." This contrasts with amino acids containing COOH or NH$_2$ side chains, which are *always* anionic (RCOO$^-$) or cationic (RNH$_3^+$) at physiological pH. [By the way, *histamine* is a small molecule that has to do with allergic responses, itching, inflammation, and other processes. (You've heard of antihistamine drugs.) It is not an amino acid; don't confuse it with *histidine*.]

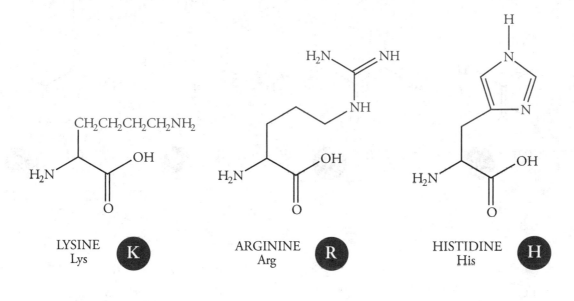

Hydrophobic (Nonpolar) Amino Acids

Hydrophobic amino acids have either aliphatic (alkyl) or aromatic side chains. Amino acids with aliphatic side chains include glycine, alanine, valine, leucine, and isoleucine. Amino acids with aromatic side chains include phenylalanine, tryptophan, and tyrosine (though the latter is a polar amino acid). Hydrophobic residues tend to associate with each other rather than with water, and therefore are found on the interior of folded globular proteins, away from water. The larger the hydrophobic group, the greater the hydrophobic force repelling it from water.

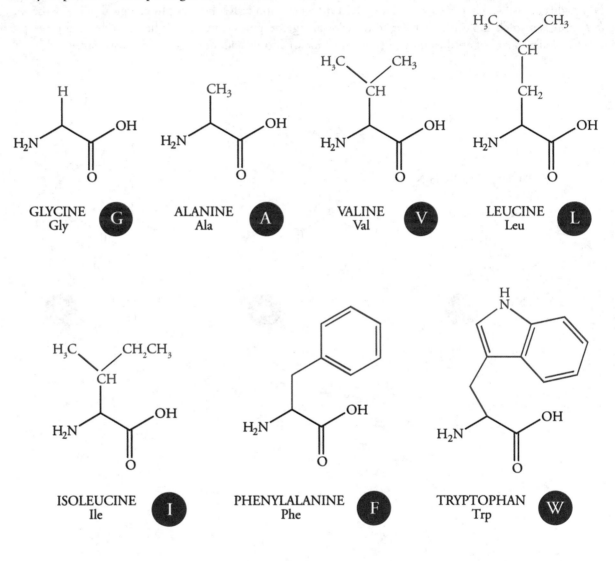

Polar Amino Acids

These amino acids are characterized by an R-group that is polar enough to form hydrogen bonds with water but which does not act as an acid or base. This means they are hydrophilic and will interact with water whenever possible. The hydroxyl groups of serine, threonine, and tyrosine residues are often modified by the attachment of a phosphate group by a regulatory enzyme called a kinase. The result is a change in structure due to the very hydrophilic phosphate group. This modification is an important means of regulating protein activity. This category also includes the amide derivatives of aspartic acid and glutamic acid, which are named asparagine and glutamine, respectively.

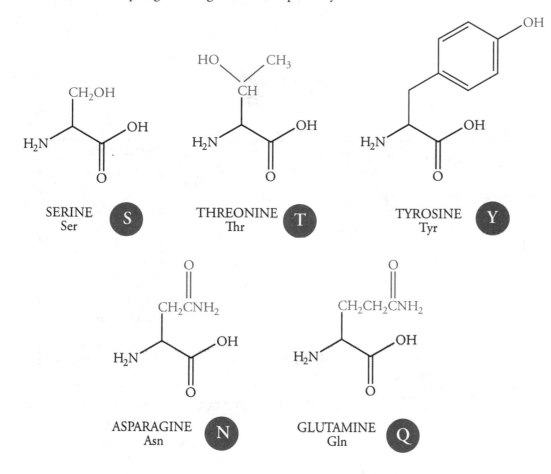

Sulfur-Containing Amino Acids

Amino acids with sulfur-containing side chains include cysteine and methionine. Cysteine, which contains a thiol (also called a sulfhydryl—like an alcohol that has an S atom instead of an O atom), is fairly polar, and methionine, which contains a thioether (like an ether that has an S atom instead of an O atom) is fairly nonpolar.

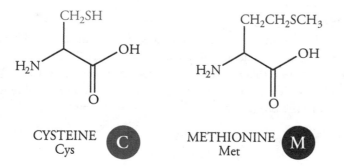

Proline

Proline is unique among the amino acids in that its amino group is covalently bound to its nonpolar side chain, creating a secondary α-amino group and a distinctive ring structure. This unique feature of proline has important consequences for protein folding (see Section 7.2).

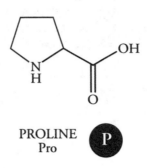

PROLINE
Pro **P**

	Hydrophilic		Hydrophobic
ACIDIC	BASIC	POLAR	NONPOLAR
Aspartic acid	Lysine*	Serine	Glycine
Glutamic acid	Arginine	Cysteine	Alanine
	Histidine*	Tyrosine	Valine*
		Threonine*	Leucine*
		Asparagine	Isoleucine*
		Glutamine	Phenylalanine*
			Tryptophan*
			Methionine*
			Proline

*Denotes one of the **nine essential** amino acids, those that cannot be synthesized by adult humans and must be obtained from the diet.

Summary Table of Amino Acids

Synthesis of Amino Acids

Nature has developed complicated mechanisms for the syntheses of the amino acids it uses to build proteins. In the laboratory, synthetic chemists have developed their own set of tools with which to make these essential building blocks available. Two important synthetic methods for the production of amino acids are the Strecker and Gabriel syntheses.

Strecker Synthesis

The Strecker synthesis utilizes ammonium and cyanide salts to transform aldehydes into α-amino acids. While naturally occurring amino acids are stereochemically pure (L-enantiomers), those produced via this process are racemic. Despite this drawback, a variety of both naturally-occurring and non-natural amino acids may be easily synthesized, depending on the substitution of the aldehyde. An example of the Strecker synthesis applied to the production of (D,L)-valine is shown below:

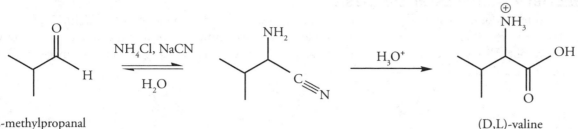

2-methylpropanal   (D,L)-valine

The combination of an ammonium halide and alkali cyanide results in the formation of alkali halide salts and the *in situ* production of the active species, NH_3 and HCN. In the first step of the reaction, the aldehyde reacts with ammonia to yield an imine as described previously in Section 6.2.

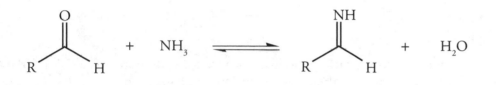

When protonated by HCN, the imine becomes more electrophilic, enabling attack by the remaining cyanide ion on the imine-carbon and concomitant formation of an α-amino nitrile. This attack by cyanide on an unsaturated carbon electrophile resembles the mechanism previously described for the formation of cyanohydrins. The difference is that the Strecker synthesis utilizes an imine (rather than a carbonyl) as substrate for the attack.

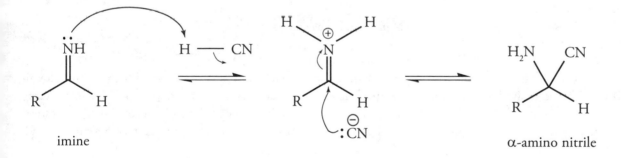

imine   α-amino nitrile

In a subsequent step, acid catalyzed hydrolysis of the α-amino nitrile gives the α-amino acid.

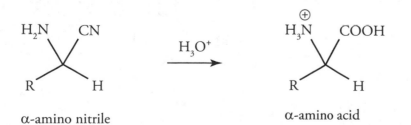

α-amino nitrile   α-amino acid

Gabriel-Malonic Ester Synthesis

The Gabriel-malonic ester synthesis is another useful method for the production of α-amino acids. Over the course of the reaction, the nitrogen in a molecule of phthalimide is converted into a primary amine. To begin, phthalimide is deprotonated with potassium hydroxide (KOH) to give the resonance-stabilized phthalimide anion, as shown below:

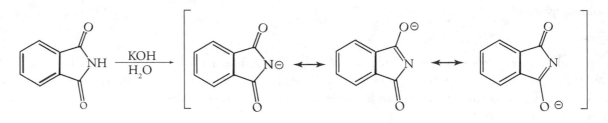

phthalimide   resonance stabilized phthalimide anion

The phthalimide anion is a strong nucleophile, and when treated with α-bromomalonic ester, it displaces bromide from the central carbon, yielding an *N*-phthalimidomalonic ester.

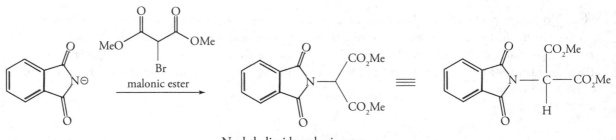

N-phthalimidomalonic ester

Enolization of the α-carbon with a strong base creates a nucleophilic carbon, which can be functional-ized with the desired amino acid side-chain. The example below shows the reaction of the enolate with methyl-(2-bromoethyl)-sulfide to give a precursor of methionine. The phthalimido group and both esters are then subjected to acid hydrolysis, and after heat-induced decarboxylation, the racemic amino acid may be isolated.

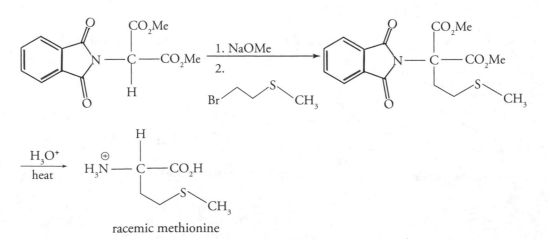

racemic methionine

Amino Acid Reactivity

Since amino acids are composed of an acidic group (the carboxylic acid) and a basic group (the amine), we must be sure to understand the acid/base chemistry of amino acids. Later, we will review amide bond formation by examining formation of the peptide bond in protein synthesis.

Reviewing the Fundamentals of Acid/Base Chemistry

Before we can discuss amino acids, we must be sure to understand the fundamentals of acid/base chemistry because each amino acid is **amphoteric**, which means it has both acidic and basic activity. This should make sense since an amino acid contains the acidic carboxylic acid group and the basic amino group.

Remember from general chemistry that acids can be defined as proton (H^+) donors, and bases can be defined as proton acceptors. Thus, in the case of the equation below, H_2A^+ is a proton donor (acid), and A^- is a proton acceptor (base); HA may act as either acid or base. The equations below also show how to calculate the equilibrium constant (K) for an acid dissociation reaction. The equilibrium constant for an acid dissociation reaction is given a special name: **acid dissociation constant**, abbreviated "K_a." The equilibrium reactions for the first and second proton dissociation reactions are described by the equations for the acid dissociation constants K_{a1} and K_{a2}.

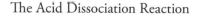

$$H_2A^+ \underset{}{\overset{(K_{a1})}{\rightleftharpoons}} HA + H^+ \underset{}{\overset{(K_{a2})}{\rightleftharpoons}} A^- + 2H^+$$

$$K_a = \frac{[products]}{[reactants]} \implies \boxed{K_{a1} = \frac{[HA]\,[H^+]}{[H_2A^+]}} \quad \boxed{K_{a2} = \frac{[A^-]\,[H^+]}{[HA]}}$$

The Acid Dissociation Reaction

2) In the equilibrium between H_2A^+, HA, and A^- above, which statement is true?[2]
   A. HA will act as a base by donating a proton.
   B. HA will act as an acid by accepting a proton.
   C. HA can act as either an acid or a base, depending on whether it accepts or donates a proton.
   D. HA is in chemical equilibrium with H_2A^+ and A^- and in that capacity cannot act as either an acid or a base.

Whether a molecule (or a functional group) is protonated depends on its affinity for protons, and the concentration of protons in solution that are available to it. Let's discuss both and do a few practice problems.

The concentration of available protons is simply $[H^+]$ (moles/liter), but it is usually expressed as **pH**, defined as $-\log [H^+]$. If you're wondering why pH is used instead of $[H^+]$, it has to do with the fact that $[H^+]$ values tend to be clumsy numbers, so a logarithmic scale reduces the amount of writing we have to do; we use the *negative* logarithm simply to avoid writing an extra minus sign. For example, instead of writing "$[H^+] = 10^{-3.46}$," we can write "pH = 3.46." The pH inside cells is 7.4. This is often referred to as **physiological pH**, and is carefully regulated by buffers in the blood because extremes of pH disrupt protein structure.

---

[2] Choice **C** is correct: In the equilibrium shown, HA can either act as an acid by donating a proton (choice B is wrong) or as a base by accepting a proton (choice A is wrong). Remember also that equilibrium is not a fixed state; in other words, HA is not doomed to stay HA forever, it can move forward and back between the states shown (choice D is wrong).

The affinity of a functional group (such as an amino or carboxyl group) for protons is given by the acid dissociation constant K_a for that functional group, which is simply the equilibrium constant for the dissociation of the acid form (HA) into a proton (H⁺) plus the conjugate base (A⁻). The equilibrium constant describes a reaction's tendency to move right or left as it moves toward equilibrium from some starting point. This affinity can also be expressed as pK_a, defined as $-\log K_a$. Carboxyl groups of amino acids generally have a pK_a of about 2 (stronger acid), while the ammonium groups generally have a pK_a of 9 or 10 (weaker acid).

The mathematical formula that describes the relationship between pH, pK_a, and the position of equilibrium in an acid-base reaction is known as the **Henderson–Hasselbalch** equation:

$$pH = pK_a + \log \frac{[A^-]}{[HA]} = pK_a + \log \frac{[\text{base form}]}{[\text{acid form}]}$$

Given the pH and the pK_a, we can calculate the ratio of the base and acid forms of a compound at equilibrium. Just remember these rules:

- Low pH means high [H⁺].
- Lower pK_a (same as higher K_a) describes a stronger acid that can donate a proton even when there are already excess protons (high [H⁺], low pH).

3) The text above states that physiological pH is 7.4. Is this more or less acidic—and are there more or fewer extra protons—than in pure water?[3]

4) Pure water at 25°C has a balance of 10^{-7} M H⁺ and 10^{-7} M OH⁻ resulting from the spontaneous breakdown of water itself. What pH does pure water have?[4]

5) What is the pH of a solution of 0.1 M HCl (assuming the HCl dissociates fully)?[5]

6) Acetic acid (CH_3COOH) has $pK_a = 4.7$. Calculate the equilibrium ratio of [CH_3COO^-] to [CH_3COOH] at pH 4.7.[6]

7) Which functional group on amino acids has a stronger tendency to donate protons: carboxyl groups ($pK_a = 2.0$) or ammonium groups ($pK_a = 9$)? Which group will donate protons at the lowest pH?[7]

---

[3] Remember that a larger pH implies *fewer* extra protons, since pH = $-\log$[H⁺]. A pH of 7.4 describes a solution with slightly fewer extra free protons, i.e., a slightly less acidic (more basic) solution, relative to a pH 7.0 solution.

[4] Simply use the formula for pH. Pure water has a pH of $-\log (10^{-7}) = 7$.

[5] The solution will have a proton concentration equal to 0.1 or 10^{-1} M. The pH of a solution with [H⁺] = 10^{-1} M is determined by the formula for pH: pH = $-\log(10^{-1} M) = 1$.

[6] First, substitute into the equation: $4.7 = 4.7 + \log$ [CH_3COO^-]/[CH_3COOH]. Then, solve:
$0 = \log$ [CH_3COO^-]/[CH_3COOH].
What has a log of 0? In other words, ten to the power of 0 is equal to what?
$10^0 = $ [CH_3COO^-]/[CH_3COOH] = 1.0
So when the pH = pK_a, the ratio of base to acid is 1 to 1. That's a fact worth memorizing.

[7] A higher pK_a means that a higher proportion of the protonated form is present relative to the unprotonated form, according to the H-H equation. High pK_a indicates a weak acid. Acids with low pK_as, tend to deprotonate more easily. Therefore, ammonium groups have a stronger tendency to keep their protons and carboxyl groups will donate protons at the lowest pH (highest [H⁺]).

Application of Fundamental Acid/Base Chemistry to Amino Acids

With that review of acids and bases, we are now prepared to discuss amino acid reactivity. The review is important because all amino acids contain an amino group that acts as a base and a carboxyl group ($pK_a \approx 2$) that acts as an acid. In its protonated, or acidic form, the amine is called an **ammonium group**, and has a pK_a between 9-10. For example:

$$-NH_3^+ \longrightarrow -NH_2 + H^+ \qquad pK_a \approx 9$$

$$-COOH \longrightarrow -COO^- + H^+ \qquad pK_a \approx 2$$

8) Assuming a pK_a of 2, will a carboxylate group be protonated or deprotonated at pH 1.0?[8]
9) Will the amino group be protonated or deprotonated at pH 1.0?[9]
10) Glycine is the simplest amino acid, with only hydrogen as its R-group. Its only functional groups are the backbone groups discussed above (amino and carboxyl). What will be the net charge on a glycine molecule at pH 12?[10]
11) At pH 6.0, between the pK_as of the ammonium and carboxyl groups, what will be the net charge on a molecule of glycine?[11]

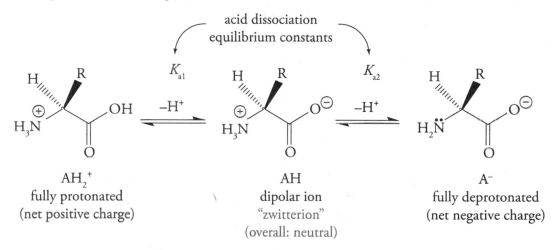

Important Amino Acid Conjugate Acid/Base Pairs

The Isoelectric Point of Amino Acids

There is a pH for every amino acid at which it has no overall net charge (the positive and negative charges cancel). A molecule with positive and negative charges that balance is referred to as a dipolar ion or **zwitterion**. The pH at which a molecule is uncharged (zwitterionic) is referred to as its **isoelectric point** (pI). "Zwitter" is German for "hybrid", implying that an amino acid at its pI has both (+) and (−) charges.

---

[8] The pH is less than the pK_a here, so protonation wins over dissociation, and the group will be protonated. The correct answer is −COOH.

[9] The pH is much lower than the pK_a for the ammonium group, so the amino group is protonated: NH_3^+.

[10] Since pH 12 represents a very low [H^+], both groups will become deprotonated (COO$^-$ and NH$_2$), creating a net charge of −1 per glycine molecule.

[11] The carboxyl group will be deprotonated (COO$^-$) with a charge of −1 and the amino group will be protonated (NH$_3^+$) with a charge of +1, creating a net charge of 0 per glycine molecule.

It is possible to calculate the pI of an amino acid—in other words, to figure out the pH value at which (+) and (–) charges balance (that's the definition of pI). For a molecule with two functional groups, such as glycine, the calculation is simple: just *average the pK_a s of the two functional groups*. The pI of more complex molecules can also be calculated, but the math is complex. For the MCAT, you should know how to calculate the pI of a molecule with two functional groups (with no acidic or basic functional groups in the side chain). Another important thing to know for the MCAT is how to compare the pH of a solution to the pK_a of a functional group of an amino acid and determine if a site is mostly protonated or deprotonated. If the pH is higher than the pK_a, the site is mostly deprotonated; if the pH is lower than the pK_a, the site is mostly protonated. This can be illustrated in the titration curve for glycine:

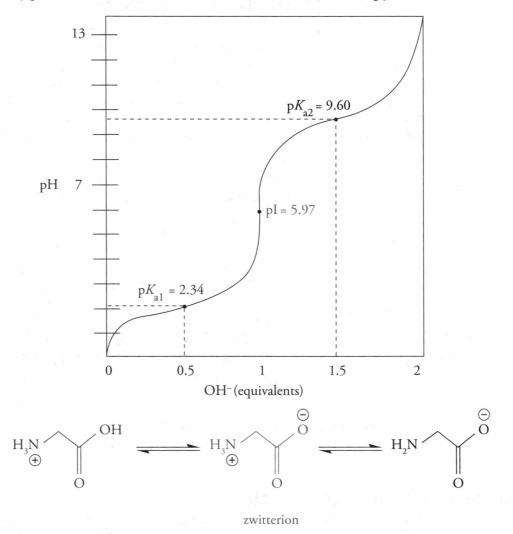

zwitterion

12) What is the pI of glycine?[12]

---

[12] To calculate the pI, just average the pK_as of the two functional groups: (9.60 + 2.34)/2 = 5.97, or roughly 6.

Amino Acid Separation—Gel Electrophoresis

Gel electrophoresis is a general separation technique that can be used to separate amino acids based on their charge. In general, when employing this technique, amino acids are loaded onto a gel that is held at a constant pH, then exposed to an electric field. When the pH of the gel is different than the pI of the amino acids, each amino acid will bear an overall charge because pI is specific to the unique structure of the side chain of each amino acid. The amino acids will therefore migrate through the gel based on their charge and the external electric field. The MCAT tends to ask about how specific amino acids will migrate relative to each other in these separation conditions. In order to answer these questions, an understanding of the relationship between pH, pK_a, and pI (as discussed previously) is required. See the table below, which summarizes how pH will determine the direction of amino acid migration during an electrophoresis separation:

pH	Charge on Amino Acid	Direction of Migration
greater than pI	negative	toward positive electrode
lower than pI	positive	toward negative electrode
equal to pI	neutral (zwitterion)	no migration

13) A sample of glycine is loaded on a gel in a pH = 6.0 solution with a (+) electrode at one end and a (–) electrode at the other end. Will the majority of the glycine migrate toward the negative terminal, migrate toward the positive terminal, or not migrate in either direction?[13]

14) The pK_as for the three functional groups in aspartic acid are 9.8 for the amino group, 2.1 for the α–carboxyl, and 3.9 for the side chain carboxyl. What pole (– or +) will aspartic acid migrate toward in an electric field at physiological pH (7.4)?[14]

15) What pole (– or +) would aspartic acid migrate toward in an electric field in a pH 1.0 solution?[15]

16) Which of these amino acids is most likely to be found on the interior of a protein at pH 7.0?[16]
   A. Alanine
   B. Glutamic acid
   C. Phenylalanine
   D. Glycine

17) Which of the following amino acids is most likely to be found on the exterior of a protein at pH 7.0?[17]
   A. Leucine
   B. Alanine
   C. Serine
   D. Isoleucine

---

[13] At this pH level, glycine has a net charge of zero. Hence, it will not move in an electric field.

[14] The amino group will be protonated ($-NH_3^+$), and both carboxyl groups deprotonated ($-COO^-$), producing an average charge per aspartic acid molecule of –1. Thus, aspartic acid will migrate toward the oppositely charged (+) pole at pH 7.4.

[15] Both carboxyl groups would be protonated and uncharged ($-COOH$), and the amino group would be protonated and charged ($-NH_3^+$). The net charge is +1, so aspartic acid would migrate toward the (–) pole.

[16] Glu is incorrect, since this amino acid is charged at a pH of 7. Of the three remaining, phenylalanine has the largest hydrophobic group, and is therefore the most likely to be found on the interior of a protein. The answer is **C**.

[17] Leucine, alanine, and isoleucine are all hydrophobic residues more likely to be found on the interior than the exterior of proteins. Serine (choice **C**), which has a hydroxyl group that can hydrogen bond with water, is the correct answer.

7.2 PROTEINS

There are two common types of covalent bonds between amino acids in proteins: the **peptide bonds** that link amino acids together into polypeptide chains and **disulfide bridges** between cysteine R-groups.

The Peptide Bond

Polypeptides are formed by linking amino acids together in peptide bonds. A peptide bond is formed between the carboxyl group of one amino acid and the α-amino group of another amino acid with the loss of water. This occurs by the same nucleophilic addition-elimination mechanism shown in Section 6.4 for formation of any one of the carboxylic acid derivatives from any other carboxylic acid derivative. Remember that a peptide bond is just an amide bond between two amino acids. The figure below shows the formation of a dipeptide from the amino acids glycine and alanine.

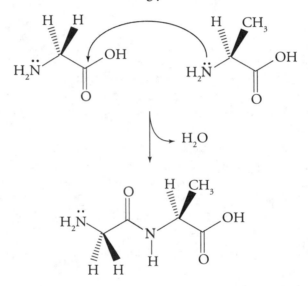

Peptide Bond (Amide Bond) Formation

Note: The above diagram showing formation of a peptide bond via a simple condensation reaction is not entirely accurate. As seen in the following graph, the formation of a peptide bond with two amino acids is not thermodynamically favorable and requires energy. This naturally occurring reaction, which takes place during translation in cells, involves enzyme catalysis, is RNA directed, and co-factor mediated.

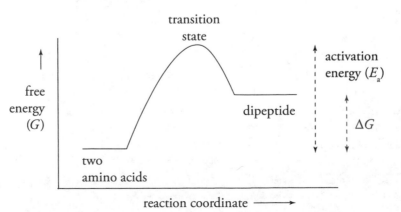

DCC Coupling

In order to synthesize peptides artificially in the laboratory, **DCC coupling** is used. In the first step of the coupling process, DCC, or dicyclohexyl carbodiimide, converts the OH of the caboxylate group in an amino acid into a good leaving group. In the next step, the amino group of a second amino acid attacks the carbonyl carbon of the "activated" amino acid. Finally, the DCC leaves with the oxygen to which it is bonded. To assure that amino acids are added in a unidirectional manner and in the proper order for the desired peptide, the reaction is run using protecting groups so that only one of the carboxyl groups and one of the amino groups are available to react. See the example reaction that follows.

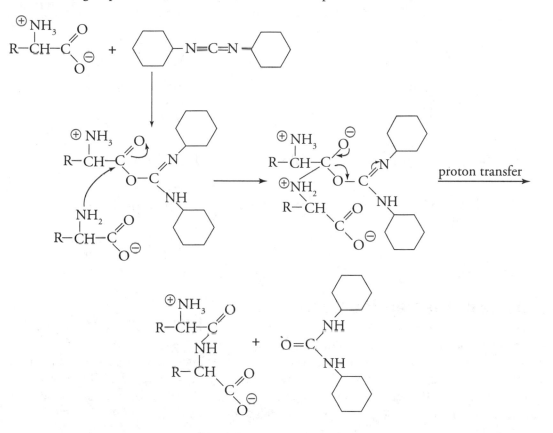

In a polypeptide chain, the N–C–C–N–C–C pattern formed from the amino acids is known as the **backbone** of the polypeptide. An individual amino acid is termed a **residue** when it is part of a polypeptide chain. The amino terminus is the first end made during polypeptide synthesis, and the carboxy terminus is made last. Hence, by convention, the amino-terminal residue is also always written first.

18) In the oligopeptide Phe-Glu-Gly-Ser-Ala, state the number of acid and base functional groups, which residue has a free α-amino group, and which residue has a free α-carboxyl group. (Refer to the beginning of the chapter for structures.)[18]

19) Thermodynamics states that free energy must decrease for a reaction to proceed spontaneously and that such a reaction will spontaneously move toward equilibrium. The reaction coordinate diagram above shows the free energy changes during peptide bond formation. At equilibrium, which is thermodynamically favored: the dipeptide or the individual amino acids?[19]

---

[18] As stated above, the amino end is always written first. Hence, the oligopeptide begins with an exposed Phe amino group and ends with an exposed Ala carboxyl; all the other backbone groups are hitched together in peptide bonds. Out of all the R-groups, there is only one acidic or basic functional group, the acidic glutamate R-group. This R-group plus the two terminal backbone groups gives a total of three acid/base functional groups.

[19] The dipeptide has a higher free energy, so its existence is less favorable. In other words, existence of the chain is less favorable than existence of the isolated amino acids.

20) In that case, how are peptide bonds formed and maintained inside cells?[20]

Planarity of the Peptide Bond

The peptide bond is planar and rigid because the resonance delocalization of the nitrogen's electrons to the carbonyl oxygen gives substantial double bond character to the bond between the carbonyl carbon and the nitrogen, as shown below. Hence there can be no rotation around the peptide bond.

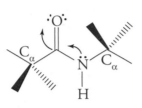

This resonance keeps the bond planar and prevents rotation.

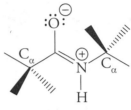

Resonance Structure of the Planar, Rigid Peptide Bond

21) If the peptide bond is rigid and planar, then is the entire polypeptide rigid and incapable of rotation?[21]

Hydrolysis of the Peptide Bond

Hydrolysis refers to any reaction in which water is inserted in a bond to cleave it. We have already discussed the details of hydrolysis reactions in Chapter 6, which covered the hydrolysis of an ester under both acidic and basic reaction conditions (see Section 6.3). Hydrolysis of the peptide bond (amide bond) to form a free amine and a carboxylic acid is thermodynamically favored (products have lower free energy), but kinetically slow. There are two common means of accelerating the rate of peptide bond hydrolysis (i.e., two common ways to destroy proteins): strong acids and proteolytic enzymes.

Acid hydrolysis is the cleaving of a protein into its constituent amino acids with strong acid and heat. This is a non-specific means of cleaving peptide bonds. The amount of each amino acid present after hydrolysis can then be quantified to determine the overall amino acid content of the protein.

22) If a tripeptide of Gly-Phe-Ala is subjected to acid hydrolysis, can the order of the residues in the tripeptide be determined afterward?[22]

---

[20] During protein synthesis, stored energy is used to force peptide bonds to form. Once the bond is formed, even though its destruction is thermodynamically favorable, it remains stable because the activation energy for the hydrolysis reaction is so high. In other words, hydrolysis is thermodynamically favorable but kinetically slow.

[21] No, only the peptide bond (between amino acids) is rigid due to resonance. The bonds to the α-carbon (within each amino acid) are free to rotate.

[22] No. After hydrolysis all amino acids are separate and have free amino and carboxyl groups.

Hydrolysis of a protein by another protein is called **proteolysis** or **proteolytic cleavage**, and the protein that does the cutting is known as a **proteolytic enzyme** or **protease**. Proteolytic cleavage is a specific means of cleaving peptide bonds. Many enzymes only cleave the peptide bond adjacent to a specific amino acid. For example, the protease trypsin cleaves on the carboxyl side of the positively charged (basic) residues arginine and lysine, while chymotrypsin cleaves adjacent to hydrophobic residues such as phenyl-alanine. (Do *not* memorize these examples.)

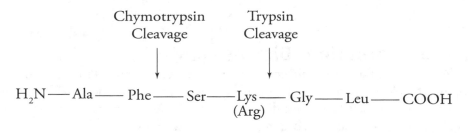

Specificity of Protease Cleavage

23) Based on the above, if the following peptide is cleaved by trypsin, what amino acid will be on the new N-terminus and how many fragments will result: Ala-Gly-Glu-Lys-Phe-Phe-Lys?[23]

The Disulfide Bond

Cysteine is an amino acid with a reactive thiol (sulfhydryl, SH) in its side chain. The thiol of one cysteine can react with the thiol of another cysteine to produce a covalent sulfur-sulfur bond known as a disulfide bond, as illustrated below. The cysteines forming a disulfide bond may be located in the same or different polypeptide chain(s). The disulfide bridge plays an important role in stabilizing tertiary protein structure; this will be discussed in the section on protein folding. Once a cysteine residue becomes disulfide-bonded to another cysteine residue, it is called *cystine* instead of cysteine.

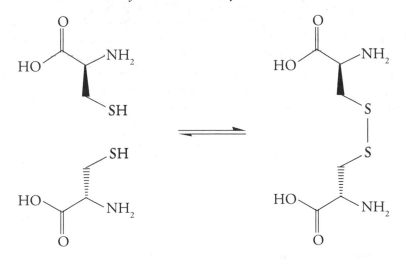

Formation of the Disulfide Bond

---

[23] Trypsin will cleave on the carboxyl side of the Lys residue, with Phe on the N-terminus of the new Phe-Phe-Lys fragment. There will be two fragments after trypsin cleavage: Phe-Phe-Lys and Ala-Gly-Glu-Lys.

24) Which is more oxidized, the sulfur in *cysteine* or the sulfur in *cystine*?[24]
25) The inside of cells is known as a reducing environment because cells possess antioxidants (chemicals that prevent oxidation reactions). Where would disulfide bridges be more likely to be found, in extracellular proteins, under oxidizing conditions, or in the interior of cells, in a reducing environment?[25]

Protein Structure in Three Dimensions

Each protein folds into a unique three-dimensional structure that is required for that protein to function properly. Improperly folded, or **denatured**, proteins are non-functional. There are four levels of protein folding that contribute to their final three-dimensional structure. Each level of structure is dependent upon a particular type of bond, as discussed in the following sections.

Denaturation is an important concept. It refers to the **disruption of a protein's shape without breaking peptide bonds**. Proteins are denatured by *urea* (which disrupts hydrogen bonding interactions), by *extremes of pH*, by extremes of *temperature*, and by *changes in salt concentration (tonicity)*.

Primary (1°) Structure: The Amino Acid Sequence

The simplest level of protein structure is the order of amino acids bonded to each other in the polypeptide chain. This linear ordering of amino acid residues is known as primary structure. Primary structure is the same as **sequence**. The bond which determines 1° structure is the peptide bond, simply because this is the bond that links one amino acid to the next in a polypeptide.

Secondary (2°) Structure: Hydrogen Bonds Between Backbone Groups

Secondary structure refers to the initial folding of a polypeptide chain into shapes stabilized by hydrogen bonds between backbone NH and CO groups. Certain motifs of secondary structure are found in most proteins. The two most common are the α-helix and the β-pleated sheet.

All α-helices have the same well-defined dimensions that are depicted below with the R-groups omitted for clarity. The α-helices of proteins are always right handed, 5 angstroms in width, with each subsequent amino acid rising 1.5 angstroms. There are 3.6 amino acid residues per turn with the α-carboxyl oxygen of one amino acid residue hydrogen-bonded to the α-amino proton of an amino acid three residues away. (*Don't* memorize these numbers, but *do* try to visualize what they mean.)

---

[24] The sulfur in cysteine is bonded to a hydrogen and a carbon; the sulfur in cystine is bonded to a sulfur and a carbon. Hence, the sulfur in cystine is more oxidized.

[25] In a reducing environment, the S-S group is reduced to two SH groups. Disulfide bridges are found only in extracellular polypeptides, where they will not be reduced. Examples of protein complexes held together by disulfide bridges include antibodies and the hormone insulin.

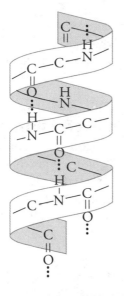

An α Helix

The unique structure of **proline** forces it to kink the polypeptide chain; hence proline residues never appear within the α-helix.

Proteins such as hormone receptors and ion channels are often found with α-helical transmembrane regions integrated into the hydrophobic membranes of cells. The α-helix is a favorable structure for a hydrophobic transmembrane region because all polar NH and CO groups in the backbone are hydrogen bonded to each other on the inside of the helix, and thus don't interact with the hydrophobic membrane interior. α-Helical regions that span membranes also have hydrophobic R-groups, which radiate out from the helix, interacting with the hydrophobic interior of the membrane.

β-Pleated sheets are also stabilized by hydrogen bonding between NH and CO groups in the polypeptide backbone. In β-sheets, however, hydrogen bonding occurs between residues distant from each other in the chain or even on separate polypeptide chains. Also, the backbone of a β-sheet is extended, rather than coiled, with side groups directed above and below the plane of the β-sheet. There are two types of β-sheets, one with adjacent polypeptide strands running in the *same* direction (**parallel** β-pleated sheet) and another in which the polypeptide strands run in *opposite* directions (**antiparallel** β-pleated sheet).

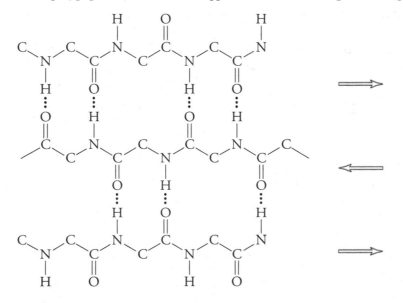

A β-Pleated Sheet

26) If a single polypeptide folds once and forms a β-pleated sheet with itself, would this be a parallel or antiparallel β-pleated sheet?[26]

27) What effect would a molecule that disrupts hydrogen bonding, e.g., urea, have on protein structure?[27]

Tertiary (3°) Structure: Hydrophobic/Hydrophilic Interactions

The next level of protein folding, tertiary structure, concerns interactions between amino acid residues located more distantly from each other in the polypeptide chain. The folding of secondary structures such as α-helices into higher order tertiary structures is driven by interactions of R-groups with each other and with the solvent (water). Hydrophobic R-groups tend to fold into the interior of the protein, away from the solvent, and hydrophilic R-groups tend to be exposed to water on the surface of the protein (shown for the generic globular protein).

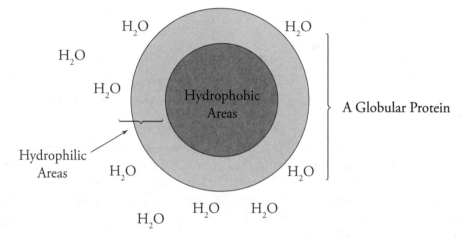

Folding of A Globular Protein in Aqueous Solution

Under the right conditions, the forces driving hydrophobic avoidance of water and hydrogen bonding will fold a polypeptide spontaneously into the correct conformation, the lowest energy conformation. In a classic experiment by Christian Anfinsen and coworkers, the effect of a denaturing agent (urea) and a reducing agent (β-mercaptoethanol) on the folding of a protein called ribonuclease were examined. In the following questions, you will reenact their thought processes. Figure out the answers before reading the footnotes.

28) Ribonuclease has eight cysteines that form four disulfides bonds. What effect would a reducing agent have on its tertiary structure?[28]

29) If the disulfides serve only to lock into place a tertiary protein structure that forms first on its own, then what effect would the reducing agent have on correct protein folding?[29]

---

[26] It would be antiparallel because one participant in the β-pleated sheet would have a C to N direction, while the other would be running N to C.

[27] Putting a protein in a urea solution will disrupt H-bonding, thus disrupting secondary structure by unfolding α-helices and β-sheets. It would not affect primary structure, which depends on the much more stable peptide bond. Disruption of 2°, 3°, or 4° structure without breaking peptide bonds is *denaturation*.

[28] The disulfide bridges would be broken. Tertiary structure would be less stable.

[29] The shape should not be disrupted if breaking disulfides is the only disturbance. It's just that the shape would be less sturdy—like a concrete wall without the rebar.

30) Would a protein end up folded normally if you (1) first put it in a reducing environment, (2) then denatured it by adding urea, (3) next removed the reducing agent, allowing disulfide bridges to reform, and (4) finally removed the denaturing agent?[30]

31) What if you did the same experiment but in this order: 1, 2, 4, 3?[31]

The disulfide bridge is perhaps not a good example of 3° structure because it is a covalent bond, not a hydrophobic interaction. However, because the disulfide is formed after 2° structure and before 4° structure, it is usually considered part of 3° folding.

32) Which of the following may be considered an example of tertiary protein structure?[32]
I. van der Waals interactions between two Phe R-groups located far apart on a polypeptide
II. Hydrogen bonds between backbone amino and carboxyl groups
III. Covalent disulfide bonds between cysteine residues located far apart on a polypeptide

33) What effect would dissolving a globular protein in a hydrophobic organic solvent such as hexane have on tertiary protein structure?[33]

Quaternary (4°) Structure: Various Bonds Between Separate Chains

The highest level of protein structure, quaternary structure, describes interactions between polypeptide subunits. A **subunit** is a single polypeptide chain that is part of a large complex containing many subunits (a **multisubunit complex**). The arrangement of subunits in a multisubunit complex is what we mean by quaternary structure. For example, mammalian RNA polymerase II contains twelve different subunits. The interactions between subunits are instrumental in protein function, as in the cooperative binding of oxygen by each of the four subunits of hemoglobin.

The forces stabilizing quaternary structure are generally the same as those involved in secondary and tertiary structure—non-covalent interactions (the hydrogen bond and the van der Waals interaction). However, covalent bonds may also be involved in quaternary structure. For example, antibodies (immune system molecules) are large protein complexes with disulfide bonds holding the subunits together. It is key to understand, however, that there is one covalent bond that may not be involved in quaternary structure—the peptide bond—because this bond defines sequence (1° structure).

34) What is the difference between a disulfide bridge involved in quaternary structure and one involved in tertiary structure?[34]

---

[30] No. If you allow disulfide bridges to form while the protein is still denatured, it will become locked into an abnormal shape.

[31] You should end up with the correct structure. In step one, you break the reinforcing disulfide bridges. In step two, you denature the protein completely by disrupting H-bonds. In step four, you allow the H-bonds to reform; as stated in the text, normally the correct tertiary structure will form spontaneously if you leave the polypeptide alone. In step three, you reform the disulfide bridges, thus locking the structure into its correct form.

[32] This is a simple question provided to clarify the classification of the disulfide bridge. Item I is a good example of 3° structure. Item II is describes 2°, not 3°, structure. Item III describes the disulfide, which is considered to be tertiary because of when it is formed, despite the fact that it is a covalent bond.

[33] The protein would be turned inside out.

[34] Quaternary disulfides are bonds that form between chains that aren't linked by peptide bonds. Tertiary disulfides are bonds that form between residues in the same polypeptide.

7.3 CARBOHYDRATES

Carbohydrates are chains of hydrated carbon atoms with the molecular formula $C_nH_{2n}O_n$. The chain usually begins with an aldehyde or ketone and continues as a polyalcohol in which each carbon has a hydroxyl substituent. Carbohydrates are produced by photosynthesis in plants and by biochemical synthesis in animals. Carbohydrates can be broken down to CO_2 in a process called **oxidation**, which is also known as burning or combustion. Because this process releases large amounts of energy, carbohydrates serve as the principle energy source for cellular metabolism. Glucose in the form of the polymer cellulose is also the building block of wood and cotton. Understanding the nomenclature, structure, and chemistry of carbohydrates is essential to understanding cellular metabolism. This chapter will also help you understand key facts such as why we can eat potatoes and cotton candy but not wood and cotton T-shirts, and why milk makes some adults flatulent.

Structure and Nomenclature of Monosaccharides

A single carbohydrate molecule is a **monosaccharide** (meaning "single sweet unit"), also known as a **simple sugar**. Two monosaccharides bonded together form a **disaccharide**; several bonded together make an **oligosaccharide**, and many make a **polysaccharide**. If these polymers are subjected to strong acid, they are hydrolyzed to monosaccharides, which are not further hydrolyzed.

Classes of monosaccharides are given a two-part name. The first part is either "aldo" or "keto," depending on whether an aldehyde or a ketone is present. The second part reveals the number of carbon atoms in the chain: trioses are the smallest and have three carbons; tetroses have four, pentoses five, hexoses six, and heptoses seven. For example, the *polyhydroxy aldehyde glucose* is an *aldohexose* because it is a six-carbon chain beginning in an aldehyde. "Glucose" and "fructose" are examples of **common names**. IUPAC nomenclature is not usually used with individual carbohydrates because the systematic names are so long.

The carbons in monosaccharides are numbered beginning with carbon #1 at the *most oxidized end* of the carbon chain, which is the end with the aldehyde or ketone.

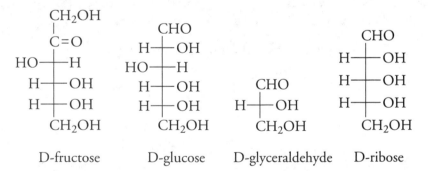

Some Metabolically Important Simple Sugars and Common Sugars on the MCAT

35) Which of the sugars in the figure above is a ketohexose?[35]
36) Which carbon (#?) is the most oxidized in fructose?[36]

---

[35] Fructose. It has six carbons, making it a hexose, and the carbonyl group is located on carbon #2, making it a ketose. Fructose is a polyhydroxy ketone, or a ketohexose.

[36] Carbon #2.

Absolute Configuration of Monosaccharides

Because carbohydrates contain chiral carbons, it is also necessary to classify them according to stereochemistry. Like amino acids, carbohydrates are assigned one of two configurations, either D or L, based on the configuration of the last chiral carbon in the chain (farthest from the aldehyde or ketone). By convention, this configuration is determined by comparison with glyceraldehyde. If a monosaccharide's last chiral carbon matches the chiral carbon of D-glyceraldehyde, it will be assigned the "D" label. The sugars in our bodies have the D configuration. When you are drawing a Fischer projection of a monosaccharide, put the aldehyde or ketone on top and the CH_2OH group (last carbon) on the bottom. The last chiral carbon will have its OH on the Left for L monosaccharides. However, we have only D-sugars in our bodies. Remember that we have only L-amino acids and only D-sugars.

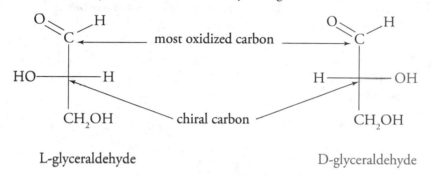

The Fischer Notation for Carbohydrates

For a given class of monosaccharide (like any other chiral molecule), there are 2^n different stereoisomers, where n is the number of chiral carbons.

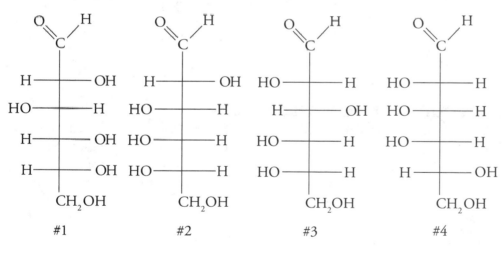

Four Monosaccharide Stereoisomers

37) Consider the four monosaccharides on the previous page. Which one of the following is correct?[37]
   A. Carbohydrate #2 is a D sugar and an enantiomer of #4.
   B. Carbohydrate #2 is an enantiomer of #3.
   C. Carbohydrates #1 and #3 are epimers and enantiomers.
   D. Carbohydrates #1 and #3 are enantiomers.

38) There are __ aldohexoses and __ D-aldohexoses (tough question but you *do* have all the information you need to figure it out).[38]

39) Is it possible to produce a diastereomer of D-glyceraldehyde? How about an epimer?[39]

Since we already discussed the relationships between the terms *isomer, stereoisomer, enantiomer, diastereomer,* and *epimer* in Chapter 4, we will not discuss them again here. The following Venn diagram represents a concise way of categorizing these terms. It shows which groups are subsets of which. *Isomers* have the same atoms but different bonds, unless they are also stereoisomers. Stereoisomers have the same atoms and the same bonds, but different bond geometries. All stereoisomers are either enantiomers or diastereomers. Some diastereomers are epimers.

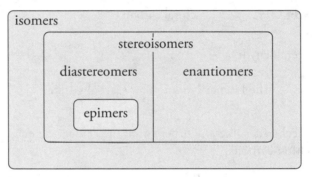

A Venn Diagram for Stereoisomers

Cyclic Structures of Monosaccharides

So far, we have represented the monosaccharides as straight chain structures. In solution, however, hexoses and pentoses spontaneously form five- and six-membered rings. In fact, the cyclic structures are thermodynamically favored, so that only a small percentage usually exist in the open chain form. The six-membered ring structures are termed **pyranoses** due to their resemblance to pyran, and five-membered sugar rings are termed **furanoses** due to their resemblance to furan.

---

[37] Sugar #2 is an L sugar, since the last chiral OH is on the left (choice A is false and can be eliminated). Sugars #2 and #3 are not mirror images, so they cannot be enantiomers (choice B is false and can be eliminated). Since sugars #1 and #3 are non-superimposable images, the are enantiomers (choice D is the correct statement), and remember that epimers are never enantiomers (choice C is false and can be eliminated).

[38] There are 2^4 aldohexoses, because there are 4 chiral carbons (#2, 3, 4, and 5). There are only 2^3 D-aldohexoses, because when you specify the "D" configuration, you leave only 3 variable chiral centers.

[39] No, it is not possible to make a glyceraldehyde diastereomer, because the molecule has only one chiral carbon. The only stereoisomer of D-glyceraldehyde is L-glyceraldehyde, an enantiomer. You can't make an epimer because the word "epimer" is reserved for sugars with more than one chiral center.

Pyran   Furan

Let's take glucose as an example. The ring forms when the OH on C5 nucleophilically attacks the carbonyl carbon (C1), forming a **hemiacetal**. The reactions involved, in which an alcohol reacts with an aldehyde to produce a hemiacetal (one −OR group and one −OH group) and subsequently an acetal (two −OR groups), are shown below (see also Section 6.2). The difference between an acetal and a hemiacetal is that the hemiacetal is in constant equilibrium with the carbonyl form. The acetal form, in contrast, is quite stable, requiring an enzyme to react.

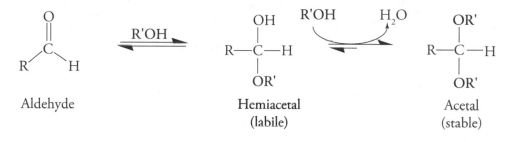

Formation of a Hemiacetal and an Acetal

The figure below shows the reaction for glucose. This manner of drawing ring structures is a modified form of Fischer notation, useful for indicating which carbons are involved in forming the cyclical structure, but unrealistic in terms of bond lengths and angles.

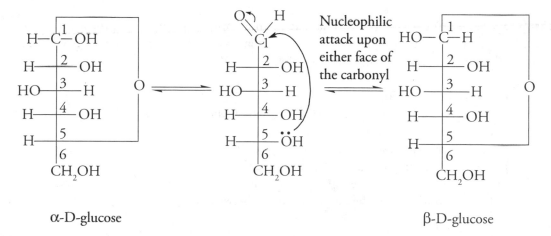

Glucopyranose Formation: A Nucleophilic Addition Reaction

The more realistic "chair" representations of these structures are shown on the next page. Note that two different ring structures are shown, α and β. The α or β ring is formed depending upon from which face of the carbonyl the C5-hydroxyl group attacks. If the attack comes from one face, the carbonyl oxygen will become an equatorial hydroxyl group; if the attack comes from the other face, the carbonyl oxygen will become an axial hydroxyl group. [To distinguish the forms, remember, "It's always better to βE up (happy)!" This will help you remember that in β-D-Glucose, the anomeric hydroxyl group is up.] The two forms are called **anomers**, and C1 (designated with an asterisk in the figures) is called the **anomeric carbon**. The anomeric carbon is always the carbonyl carbon, so in aldoses it is C1, but in ketoses it is C2. The interconversion between the two anomers is called **mutarotation**.

The groups on the *left* in Fischer notation are *above* the ring in chair notation. Also, remember that *axial* substituents on six-membered chair rings are those that point *straight up or down*. The *equatorial* substituents point *out* from the ring. Equatorial substituents have less steric hindrance with the ring and are thus thermodynamically more favorable.

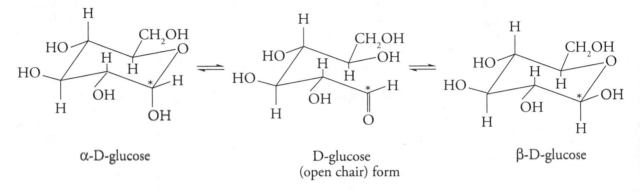

α-D-glucose   D-glucose (open chair) form   β-D-glucose

Chair Representation of Glucopyranose Formation

40) Why doesn't glucose cyclize into three- or four-membered rings?[40]
41) Are the OH's in β-D-glucopyranose axial or equatorial?[41]
42) A solution of glucose may contain both furanose and pyranose rings. How can the same sugar exist in both forms?[42]

Another way to represent cyclic sugars is called Haworth notation. The groups on the *left* in Fischer notation are *above* the ring in Haworth notation (as in the chair form). A summary of how to convert Fischer Projections of sugars to Haworth Projections is as follows:

1. Draw the basic structure of the sugar.
2. If the sugar is a D-sugar, place a –CH$_2$OH above the ring on the carbon to the left of the oxygen. For an L-sugar, place it below the ring.
3. For an α-sugar, place an –OH below the ring on the carbon to the right of the ring oxygen. For a β-sugar, place the –OH above the ring.
4. Finally, –OH groups on the right go below the ring and those on the left above, using the –CH$_2$OH group as the reference point for both projections.

---

[40] Smaller rings necessitate bond angles that are much narrower than the normal tetrahedral angle. Strained bonds are unfavorable because they are high energy.

[41] They are all equatorial. This makes it a very stable molecule, and may explain why it is the most prevalent sugar in nature. It stores a lot of energy, and yet is very stable. (Key fact.)

[42] The structure that forms depends on which OH attacks the carbonyl carbon (C#1). If OH4 attacks the carbonyl, the result will be a five-membered ring. If OH5 attacks, the result will be a six-membered ring. If you actually counted the structures in solution, you'd find more six-membered rings, since these are inherently more stable due to bond angles.

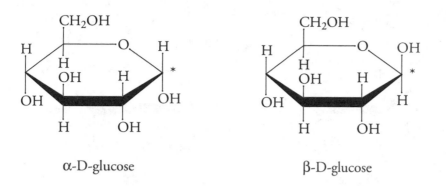

α-D-glucose   β-D-glucose

Haworth Representation of Glucopyranose

43) A monosaccharide is represented below in Haworth notation. What number is the carbon that the arrow is pointing toward? Is this a furanose or a pyranose? Is it the α- or β-anomer?[43]

44) Is this a D- or L-sugar? How many chiral carbons does it have?[44]

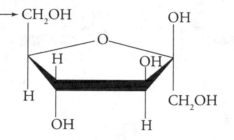

Structure and Nomenclature of Disaccharides

Recall that two monosaccharides bonded together form a disaccharide, a few form an oligosaccharide, and many form a polysaccharide. The bond between two sugar molecules is called a **glycosidic linkage**. This is a covalent bond, formed in a dehydration reaction that requires enzymatic catalysis.

Typically, the glycosidic bond joins C1 of one pyranose or furanose to C4 (sometimes C2 or C6) of another pyranose or furanose through an oxygen atom. Is the anomeric carbon in a hemiacetal form, or is it in an acetal form once it is part of a glycosidic bond? It has two –OR constituents, so it forms an acetal group. The significance of this is that the glycosidic linkage stays in the α or β configuration until an enzyme breaks the bond, because the acetal is a stable functional group. In other words, once a monosaccharide has attacked another sugar to form a glycosidic linkage, it is no longer free to mutarotate. This is an important concept, and we will discuss it further in the section on reducing sugars.

---

[43] It is the one farthest from the anomeric carbon, so it is #6. It is in a five-membered ring, so it is a furanose. The anomeric OH (former carbonyl O) is up, so it's β.

[44] It is D-fructose, with three chiral carbons (four when cyclic). One way to determine that it's a D sugar is to identify the penultimate chiral carbon, mentally open the chain, and visualize it as a Fischer structure. Another is to assign absolute configuration. D sugars have *R* configurations at the penultimate carbon.

7.3

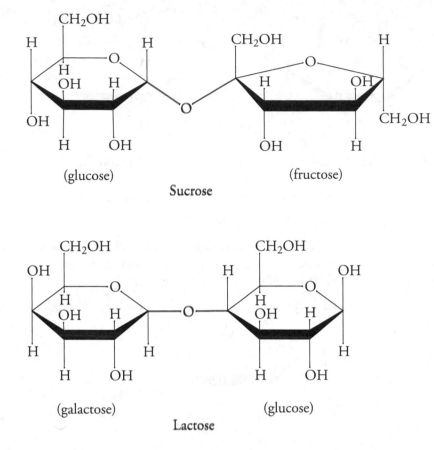

(glucose)　　　　　　　　　　(fructose)

Sucrose

(galactose)　　　　　　　　　(glucose)

Lactose

Disaccharides and the α- or β-Glycosidic Bond

Glycosidic linkages are named according to which carbon in each sugar comprises the linkage. The configuration (α or β) of the linkage is also specified. For example, lactose (milk sugar) is a disaccharide joined in a galactose-β-1,4-glucose linkage (above). Sucrose (table sugar) is also shown above, with a glucose unit and a fructose unit.

45) Does sucrose contain an α- or β-glycosidic linkage?[45]

Some common disaccharides you might see on the MCAT are sucrose (Glc-α-1,2-Fru), lactose (Gal-β-1,4-Glc), maltose (Glc-α-1,4-Glc), and cellobiose (Glc-β-1,4-Glc). However, you should NOT try to memorize these linkages.

Polymers made from these disaccharides form important biological macromolecules. Glycogen serves as an energy storage carbohydrate in animals and is composed of thousands of glucose units joined in α-1,4 linkages; α-1,6 branches are also present. Starch is the same as glycogen (except that the branches are a little different), and serves the same purpose in plants. Cellulose is a polymer of cellobiose; the β-glycosidic bonds allow the polymer to assume a long, straight, fibrous shape. Wood and cotton are made of cellulose.

---

[45] The anomeric carbon of glucose is pointing down, which means the linkage is α-1,2. So, sucrose is Glc-α-1,2-Fru.

The hydrolysis of polysaccharides into monosaccharides is essential for monosaccharides to enter metabolic pathways (e.g., glycolysis) and be used for energy by the cell. Different enzymes catalyze the hydrolysis of different linkages. The enzyme is named for the sugar it hydrolyzes. For example, the enzyme that catalyzes the hydrolysis of maltose into two glucose monosaccharides is called **maltase**. Each enzyme is highly specific for its linkage.

This specificity is a great example of the significance of stereochemistry. Consider cellulose. A cotton T-shirt is pure sugar. The only reason we can't digest it is that mammalian enzymes can't deal with the β-glycosidic linkages that make cellobiose from glucose. Cellulose is actually the energy source in grass and hay. Cows are mammals, and all mammals lack the enzymes necessary for cellobiose breakdown. To live on grass, cows depend on bacteria that live in an extra stomach called a rumen to digest cellulose for them. If you're really on the ball, you're next question is: Humans are mammals, so how can we digest lactose, which has a β linkage? The answer is that we have a specific enzyme, **lactase**, which can digest lactose. This is an exception to the rule that mammalian enzymes cannot hydrolyze β-glycosidic linkages. People without lactase are **lactose malabsorbers**, and any lactose they eat ends up in the colon. There it may cause gas and diarrhea, if certain bacteria are present; people with this problem are said to be **lactose intolerant**. People produce lactase as children so that they can digest mother's milk, but most adults naturally stop making this enzyme, and thus become lactose malabsorbers and sometimes intolerant.

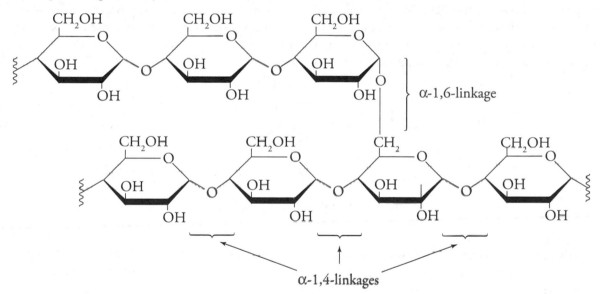

The Polysaccharide Glycogen

Hydrolysis of Glycosidic Linkages

Disaccharides and polysaccharides are broken down into their component monosaccharides by enzymatic hydrolysis. This just means water is the nucleophile, and one of the sugars is the leaving group (the one that was the attacker during bond formation). In other words, the cleavage reaction is precisely the reverse of the formation reaction.

Hydrolysis of polysaccharides into monosaccharides is favored thermodynamically. This means the hydrolysis of polysaccharides releases energy in the cell. However, it does not occur at a significant rate without enzymatic catalysis. As catalysts, enzymes increase reaction rates by lowering the activation energy but do not change final concentrations of reactants and products.

46) Which requires net energy input: polysaccharide synthesis or hydrolysis?[46]
47) If the activation energy of polysaccharide hydrolysis were so low that no enzyme was required for the reaction to occur, would this make polysaccharides better for energy storage?[47]

Reducing Sugars

This is a simple concept that often confuses students. **Benedict's test** is a chemical assay that detects the carbonyl units of sugars. It is useful because it distinguishes hemiacetals from acetals [only hemiacetals are in equilibrium with the carbonyl (open-chain) form]. For example, if you had a white powder that you knew to be composed of glucose, you would be able to say whether the glucose existed in the free monosaccharide form or was in the form of glycogen. How? Well, if it's in the monosaccharide form, there will be many hemiacetals, and Benedict's test will be strongly positive. However, if the powder consists of only relatively few glycogen molecules, Benedict's will be only weakly positive. This is because all the glucose units in a glycogen polymer are tied up in acetal linkages, except for the very first one in the chain (the one which was first attacked during polymerization).

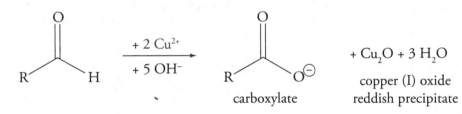

Benedict's Test for Reducing Sugars

Benedict's test is performed as follows: Benedict's reagent, an oxidized form of copper, is used to oxidize a sugar's aldehyde or ketone to the corresponding carboxylic acid, yielding a reddish precipitate. Any carbohydrate that can be oxidized by Benedict's reagent is referred to as a **reducing sugar** because it *reduces* the Cu^{2+} to Cu^+ while itself being oxidized. All monosaccharides are reducing sugars. More generally, *all aldehydes, ketones, and hemiacetals give a positive result in Benedict's test for reducing sugars; acetals give a negative result because they do not react with Cu^{2+}, and they are not in equilibrium with the open-chain (carbonyl) form.*

48) Which carbon of glucose can be oxidized by Benedict's reagent? What about fructose?[48]

---

[46] Because hydrolysis of polysaccharides is thermodynamically favored, energy input is required to drive the reaction toward polysaccharide synthesis.

[47] No, because then polysaccharides would hydrolyze spontaneously (they'd be unstable). The high activation energy of polysaccharide hydrolysis allows us to use enzymes as gatekeepers—when we need energy from glucose, we open the gate of glycogen hydrolysis.

[48] The anomeric carbon, which is #1 for aldoses like glucose and #2 for ketoses like fructose.

Recall that we've said once a monosaccharide has attacked another sugar to form a glycosidic linkage, it is no longer free to mutarotate. Now we can expand this statement as follows: Once a monosaccharide has attacked another sugar to form a glycosidic linkage, its anomeric carbon is in an acetal configuration and is thus no longer free to mutarotate *nor to reduce Benedict's reagent*.

49) If 98% of a monosaccharide is present as the ring form at equilibrium in solution, then how much of the sugar can be oxidized in Benedict's reaction?[49]
50) Is lactose a reducing sugar? What about sucrose? (You may refer back to the text and figures previously.)[50]

7.4 LIPIDS

Lipids are oily or fatty substances that play three physiological roles, summarized here and discussed below.

- In cellular membranes, phospholipids constitute a barrier between intracellular and extracellular environments.
- In adipose cells, triglycerides (fats) store energy.
- Finally, cholesterol is a special lipid that serves as the building block for the hydrophobic steroid hormones.

The cardinal characteristic of the lipid is its **hydrophobicity**. Hydrophobic means *water-fearing*. It is important to understand the significance of this. Since water is very polar, polar substances dissolve well in water; these are known as *water-loving*, or **hydrophilic** substances. Carbon-carbon bonds and carbon-hydrogen bonds are nonpolar. Hence, substances that contain only carbon and hydrogen will not dissolve well in water. Some examples: table sugar dissolves well in water, but cooking oil floats in a layer above water or forms many tiny oil droplets when mixed with water. Cotton T-shirts become wet when exposed to water because they are made of glucose polymerized into cellulose, but a nylon jacket does not become wet because it is composed of atoms covalently bound together in a nonpolar fashion. A synonym for hydrophobic is **lipophilic** (which means lipid-loving); a synonym for hydrophilic is **lipophobic**. We return to these concepts below.

Fatty Acid Structure

Fatty acids are composed of long unsubstituted alkanes that end in a carboxylic acid. The chain is typically 14 to 18 carbons long, and because they are synthesized two carbons at a time from acetate, only *even-numbered* fatty acids are made in human cells. A fatty acid with no carbon-carbon double bonds is said to be **saturated** with hydrogen because every carbon atom in the chain is covalently bound to the maximum

---

[49] 100% will be oxidized. In a monosaccharide, the ring form is in equilibrium with the open chain form. So when the open chain form is used up in the oxidation reaction, it will be replenished by other rings opening up (Le Châtelier's principle).

[50] Lactose (Gal-β-1-,4-Glc) is a reducing sugar. Although the attacking anomeric carbon becomes locked in an acetal, the anomeric carbon of the *attacked* monosaccharide is still free to mutarotate or react with Benedict's reagent. Sucrose (Glc-α-1-,2-Fru) is not a reducing sugar, because it is made of glucose and fructose, which are both joined at their anomeric carbons. Carbon #1 of glucose is the anomeric carbon, since glucose is an aldose; carbon #2 of fructose is the anomeric carbon, since fructose is a ketose.

number of hydrogens. **Unsaturated** fatty acids have one or more double bonds in the tail. These double bonds are almost always (Z) (or *cis*). The position of a double bond in the alkyl chain of a fatty acid is denoted by the symbol Δ and the number of the first carbon involved in the double bond. Carbons are numbered starting with the carboxylic acid carbon. For example, a (Z) double bond between carbons 3 and 4 in a fatty acid would be referred to as (Z)-Δ^3 (or *cis*-Δ^3).

Saturated fatty acid

Unsaturated fatty acid

51) What is the correct nomenclature for the double bond in the unsaturated fatty acid above?[51]
52) How does the shape of an unsaturated fatty acid differ from that of a saturated fatty acid?[52]
53) If fatty acids are mixed into water, how are they likely to associate with each other?[53]

The drawing on the next page illustrates how free fatty acids interact in an aqueous solution; they form a structure called a **micelle**. The force that drives the tails into the center of the micelle is called the **hydrophobic interaction**. The hydrophobic interaction is a complex phenomenon. In general, it results from the fact that water molecules must form an orderly **solvation shell** around each hydrophobic substance. The reason is that H_2O has a dipole that "likes" to be able to share its charges with other polar molecules. A solvation shell allows for the most water-water interaction and the least water-lipid interaction. The problem is that forming a solvation shell is an increase in order and thus a decrease in entropy ($\Delta S < 0$), which is unfavorable according to the second law of thermodynamics. In the case of the fatty acid micelle, water forms a shell around the spherical micelle with the result being that water interacts with polar carboxylic acid head groups while hydrophobic lipid tails hide inside the sphere.

Soaps are the sodium salts of fatty acids ($RCOO^-Na^+$). They are **amphipathic**, which means both hydrophilic and hydrophobic.

---

[51] This double bond extends between carbons 7 and 8, and is *cis*. The bond therefore is *cis*-Δ^7.

[52] An unsaturated fatty acid is bent, or "kinked," at the *cis* double bond.

[53] The long hydrophobic chains will interact with each other to minimize contact with water, exposing the charged carboxyl group to the aqueous environment.

7.4

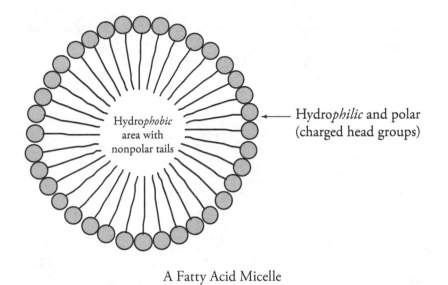

Hydro*phobic* area with nonpolar tails

⟵— Hydro*philic* and polar (charged head groups)

A Fatty Acid Micelle

54) How does soap help to remove grease from your hands?[54]

Triacylglycerols (TG)

The storage form of the fatty acid is fat. The technical name for fat is **triacylglycerol** or **triglyceride** (shown below). The triglyceride is composed of three fatty acids esterified to a glycerol molecule. Glycerol is a three-carbon triol with the formula $HOCH_2$–$CHOH$–CH_2OH. As you can see, it has three hydroxyl groups that can be esterified to fatty acids. It is necessary to store fatty acids in the relatively inert form of fat because free fatty acids are reactive chemicals.

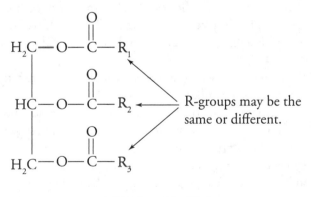

A Triglyceride (Fat)

The triacylglycerol undergoes reactions typical of esters, such as base-catalyzed hydrolysis. Soap is economically produced by base-catalyzed hydrolysis of triglycerides from animal fat into fatty acid salts (soaps). This reaction is called **saponification** and is illustrated below.

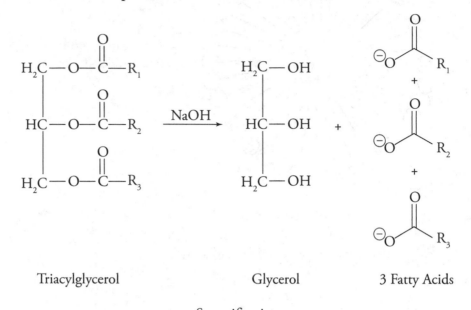

Triacylglycerol   Glycerol   3 Fatty Acids

Saponification

Lipases are enzymes that hydrolyze fats. Triacylglycerols are stored in fat cells as an energy source. Fats are more efficient energy storage molecules than carbohydrates for two reasons: packing and energy content.

> Packing: Their hydrophobicity allows fats to pack together much more closely than carbohydrates. Carbohydrates carry a great amount of water-of-solvation (water molecules hydrogen bonded to their hydroxyl groups). In other words, the amount of carbon per unit area or unit weight is much greater in a fat droplet than in dissolved sugar. If we could store sugars in a dry powdery form in our bodies, this problem would be obviated.

> Energy content: All packing considerations aside, fat molecules store much more energy than carbohydrates. In other words, regardless of what you dissolve it in, a fat has more energy carbon-for-carbon than a carbohydrate. The reason is that fats are much more *reduced*. Remember that energy metabolism begins with the *oxidation* of foodstuffs to release energy. Since carbohydrates are more oxidized to start with, oxidizing them releases less energy. Animals use fat to store most of their energy, storing only a small amount as carbohydrates (glycogen). Plants such as potatoes commonly store a large percentage of their energy as carbohydrates (starch).

Introduction to Lipid Bilayer Membranes

Membrane lipids are **phospholipids** derived from diacylglycerol phosphate or DG-P. For example, phosphatidyl choline is a phospholipid formed by the esterification of a choline molecule [$HO(CH_2)_2N^+(CH_3)_3$] to the phosphate group of DG-P. Phospholipids are **detergents**, substances that efficiently solubilize oils while remaining highly water-soluble. Detergents are like soaps, but stronger.

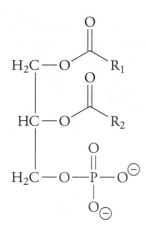

A Phosphoglyceride (Diacylglycerol Phosphate, or DGP)

We saw previously how fatty acids spontaneously form micelles. Phospholipids also minimize their interactions with water by forming an orderly structure—in this case, it is a **lipid bilayer** (below). Hydrophobic interactions drive the formation of the bilayer, and once formed, it is stabilized by van der Waals forces between the long tails.

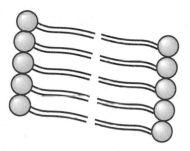

A Small Section of a Lipid Bilayer Membrane

55) Would a saturated or an unsaturated fatty acid residue have more van der Waals interactions with neighboring alkyl chains in a bilayer membrane?[55]

A more precise way to give the answer to the question above is to say that double bonds (unsaturation) in phospholipid fatty acids *tend to increase membrane fluidity*. Unsaturation prevents the membrane from solidifying by disrupting the orderly packing of the hydrophobic lipid tails. This decreases the melting point. The right amount of fluidity is essential for function. Decreasing the *length* of fatty acid tails also increases fluidity. The steroid **cholesterol** (discussed a bit later) is a third important modulator of membrane fluidity. At low temperatures, it increases fluidity in the same way as kinks in fatty acid tails; hence, it is known as membrane antifreeze. At high temperatures, however, cholesterol attenuates (reduces) membrane fluidity. Don't ponder this paradox too long; just remember that cholesterol keeps fluidity at an *optimum level*. Remember, the structural determinants of membrane fluidity are: degree of saturation, tail length, and amount of cholesterol.

---

[55] The bent shape of the unsaturated fatty acid means that it doesn't fit in as well and has less contact with neighboring groups to form van der Waals interactions. Unsaturation makes the membrane less stable, less solid.

The lipid bilayer acts like a plastic bag surrounding the cell in the sense that it seals the interior of the cell from the exterior. However, the cell membrane is much more complex than a plastic bag. Since the plasma bilayer membrane surrounding cells is impermeable to charged particles such as Na^+, protein gateways such as ion channels are required for ions to enter or exit cells. Proteins that are integrated into membranes also transmit signals from the outside of the cell into the interior. For example, certain hormones (peptides) cannot pass through the cell membrane due to their charged nature; instead, protein **receptors** in the cell membrane bind these hormones and transmit a signal into the cell in a **second messenger cascade**.

Terpenes

A terpene is a member of a broad class of compounds built from isoprene units (C_5H_8) with a general formula $(C_5H_8)_n$.

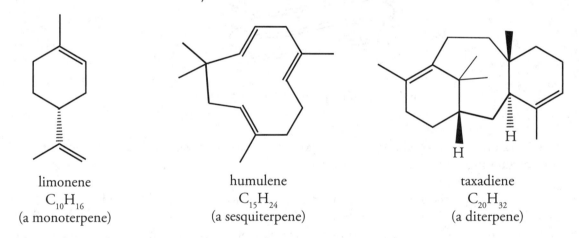

isoprene

Terpenes may be linear or cyclic, and are classified by the number of isoprene units they contain. For example, monoterpenes consist of two isoprene units, sesquiterpenes consist of three, and diterpenes contain four.

limonene
$C_{10}H_{16}$
(a monoterpene)

humulene
$C_{15}H_{24}$
(a sesquiterpene)

taxadiene
$C_{20}H_{32}$
(a diterpene)

Squalene is a triterpene (made of six isoprene units), and is a particularly important compound as it is biosynthetically utilized in the manufacture of steroids.

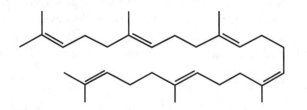

Whereas a terpene is formally a simple hydrocarbon, there are a number of natural and synthetically derived species that are built from an isoprene skeleton and functionalized with other elements (O, N, S, etc.). These functionalized-terpenes are known as *terpenoids*. Vitamin A ($C_{20}H_{30}O$) is an example of a terpenoid.

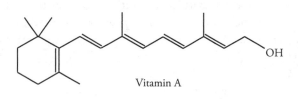

Vitamin A

Steroids

Steroids are included here because of their hydrophobicity, and, hence, similarity to fats. Their structure is otherwise unique. All steroids have the basic tetracyclic ring system (see below), based on the structure of **cholesterol**, a polycyclic amphipath. (Polycyclic means several rings, and amphipathic means displaying both hydrophilic and hydrophobic characteristics.)

As discussed above, the steroid cholesterol is an important component of the lipid bilayer. It is obtained from the diet and synthesized in the liver. It is carried in the blood packaged with fats and proteins into **lipoproteins**. One type of lipoprotein has been implicated as the cause of atherosclerotic vascular disease, which refers to the build-up of cholesterol "plaques" on the inside of blood vessels.

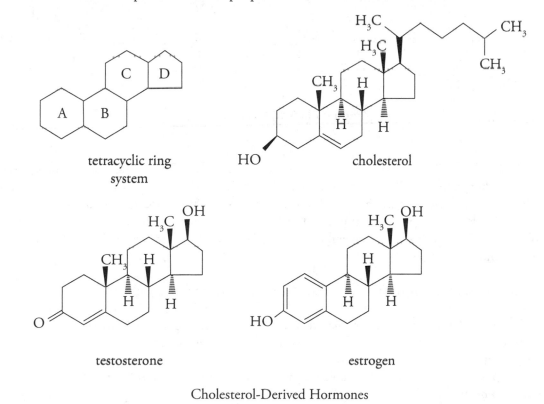

tetracyclic ring
system

cholesterol

testosterone

estrogen

Cholesterol-Derived Hormones

Steroid hormones are made from cholesterol. Two examples are **testosterone** (an androgen or male sex hormone) and **estradiol** (an estrogen or female sex hormone). There are no receptors for steroid hormones on the surface of cells. If this is true, how can they exert an influence on the cell? Because steroids are highly hydrophobic, they can diffuse right through the lipid bilayer membrane into the cytoplasm. The receptors for steroid hormones are located within cells rather than on the cell surface. This is an important point! You must be aware of the contrast between *peptide* hormones, such as insulin, which exert their effects by binding to receptors at the cell-surface, and *steroid* hormones, such as estrogen, which diffuse into cells to find their receptors.

7.5 NUCLEIC ACIDS

Before we can talk about nucleic acids, we must first briefly review some background.

Phosphorus-Containing Compounds

Phosphoric acid is an *inorganic* acid (it does not contain carbon) with the potential to donate three protons. The K_as for the three acid dissociation equilibria are 2.1, 7.2, and 12.4. Therefore, at physiological pH, phosphoric acid is significantly dissociated, existing largely in anionic form.

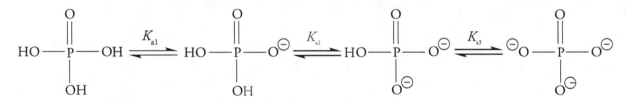

Phosphoric Acid Dissociation

Phosphate is also known as orthophosphate. Two orthophosphates bound together via an **anhydride linkage** form **pyrophosphate**. The P–O–P bond in pyrophosphate is an example of a **high-energy phosphate bond**. This name is derived from the fact that the hydrolysis of pyrophosphate is thermodynamically extremely favorable (shown on the next page). The $\Delta G°$ for the hydrolysis of pyrophosphate is about –7 kcal/mol. This means that it is a very favorable reaction. The actual $\Delta G°$ in the cell is about –12 kcal/mol, which is even more favorable.

There are three reasons that phosphate anhydride bonds store so much energy:

1. When phosphates are linked together, their negative charges repel each other strongly.
2. Orthophosphate has more resonance forms and thus a lower free energy than linked phosphates.
3. Orthophosphate has a more favorable interaction with the biological solvent (water) than linked phosphates.

The details are not crucial. What is essential is that you fix the image in your mind of linked phosphates acting like compressed springs, just waiting to fly open and provide energy for an enzyme to catalyze a reaction.

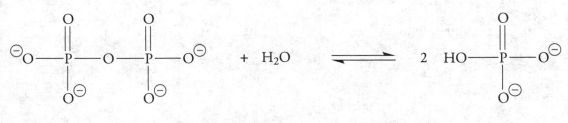

The Hydrolysis of Pyrophosphate

Nucleotides

Nucleotides are the building blocks of nucleic acids (RNA and DNA). Each nucleotide contains a **ribose** (or **deoxyribose**) **sugar** group; a purine or pyrimidine base joined to carbon number one of the ribose ring; and one, two, or three **phosphate units** joined to carbon five of the ribose ring. The nucleotide adenosine triphosphate (ATP) plays a central role in cellular metabolism in addition to being an RNA precursor.

ATP is the universal short-term energy storage molecule. Energy extracted from the oxidation of foodstuffs is immediately stored in the phosphoanhydride bonds of ATP. This energy will later be used to power cellular processes; it may also be used to synthesize glucose or fats, which are longer-term energy storage molecules. This applies to *all* living organisms, from bacteria to humans. Even some viruses carry ATP with them outside the host cell, though viruses cannot make their own ATP.

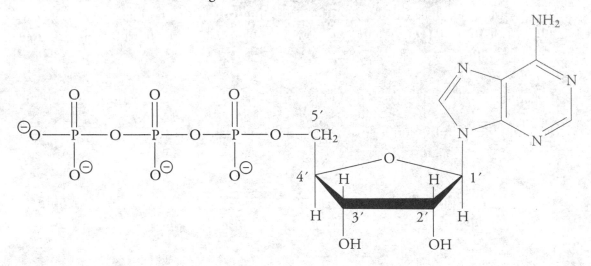

Adenosine Triphosphate (ATP)

Chapter 7 Summary

- Amino acids (AAs) consist of a tetrahedral α-carbon connected to an amino group, a carboxyl group, and a variable R group, which determines the AA's properties.

- The isoelectric point of an AA is the pH at which the net charge on the molecule is zero; this structure is referred to as the *zwitterion*.

- Electrophoresis separates mixtures of AAs and is conducted at buffered pH. Positively charged AAs move to the "−" end of the gel, and negative AAs move to the "+" end. Zwitterions will not move.

- Proteins consist of amino acids linked by peptide bonds, or amide bonds, which have partial double bond characteristics, lack rotation and are very stable.

- The secondary structure of proteins (α-helices and β-sheets) is formed through hydrogen bonding interactions between atoms in the backbone of the molecule.

- The most stable tertiary protein structure generally places polar AAs on the exterior and nonpolar AAs on the interior of the protein. This minimizes interactions between nonpolar AAs and water, while optimizing interactions between side chains inside the protein.

- All animal amino acids are L-configuration and all animal sugars are D-configuration.

- Carbohydrates are chains of hydrated carbon atoms with the molecular formula $C_nH_{2n}O_n$.

- Sugars in solution exist in equilibrium between the straight chain form and either the furanose (five-atom) or pyranose (six-atom) cyclic forms.

- The anomeric forms of a sugar differ by the position of the OH group on the anomeric carbon; OH down = α, OH up = β.

- All monosaccharides will give a positive result in a Benedict's test because they contain an aldehyde, ketone or hemiacetal, and are therefore reducing sugars.

- The glycosidic linkage in a disaccharide is named based on which anomer is present for the sugar containing the acetal and the numbers of the carbons linked to the bridging O.

- Saponification (base-mediated hydrolysis) of a triglyceride produces three equivalents of fatty acid carboxylates. These amphipathic molecules form micelles in solution.

- Lipids are found in several forms in the body, including triglycerides, phospholipids, cholesterol and steroids.

- The building blocks of nucleic acids (DNA and RNA) are nucleotides, which are comprised of a pentose sugar, a purine or pyrimidine base, and 2-3 phosphate units.

CHAPTER 7 FREESTANDING PRACTICE QUESTIONS

1. Which of the following best explains the strength of the peptide bond in a protein?

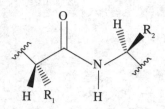

A) The steric bulk of the R groups prevents nucleophilic attack at the carbonyl carbon.
B) The electron pair on the nitrogen atom is delocalized by orbital overlap with the carbonyl group.
C) Peptide bonds are never exposed to the exterior of a protein.
D) The peptide bond is resistant to hydrolysis by many biological molecules.

2. Why is ATP known as a "high energy" structure at neutral pH?

A) It exhibits a large decrease in free energy when it undergoes hydrolytic reactions.
B) The phosphate ion released from ATP hydrolysis is very reactive.
C) It causes cellular processes to proceed at faster rates.
D) Adenine is the best energy storage molecule of all the nitrogenous bases.

3. Which of the following best describes the secondary structure of a protein?

A) Various folded polypeptide chains joining together to form a larger unit
B) The amino acid sequence of the chain
C) The polypeptide chain folding upon itself due to hydrophobic/hydrophilic interactions
D) Peptide bonds hydrogen-bonding to one another to create a sheet-like structure

4. Which of the following fatty acids has the highest melting point?

A) 4,5-Dimethylhexanoic acid
B) Octanoic acid
C) 2,3-Dimethylbutanoic acid
D) Hexanoic acid

5. Which of the following terms best describes the interconversion between α-D-glucose and β-D-glucose?

A) Tautomerism
B) Nucleophilic addition
C) Mutarotation
D) Elimination

6. A dipeptide is synthesized with the sequence Asp-Glu. The aspartic acid residue has an observed pK_a of 2.10 for its side chain. In free glutamic acid, the side chain has an expected pK_a of 2.15. However, in this dipeptide, it is likely that the observed pK_a of the glutamic acid side chain will be:

A) higher due to a favorable ionic interaction between the deprotonated side chains.
B) lower due to a favorable ionic interaction between the deprotonated side chains.
C) higher due to an unfavorable ionic interaction between the deprotonated side chains.
D) lower due to an unfavorable ionic interaction between the deprotonated side chains.

7. In the dipeptide shown below, all of the labeled dihedral angles may freely rotate EXCEPT:

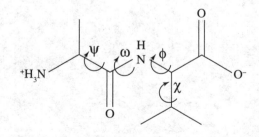

A) ω
B) ψ
C) χ
D) φ

CHAPTER 7 PRACTICE PASSAGE

In the body, proteins are constantly being synthesized and degraded in order to maintain and modulate protein concentration and enzyme activity levels. In eukaryotic cells, a 76-residue protein called *ubiquitin* is used as a tag to label proteins destined for degradation.

Ubiquitin forms an amide bond between its glycine residue at position 76 and the side chain of a lysine residue of the target protein. Three enzymes are required in the attachment of ubiquitin to the target protein. The steps of ubiquitination at pH 7 are shown in Figure 1. The first step is coupled to ATP hydrolysis.

First, a single ubiquitin is attached to the target protein via the reaction shown in Figure 1. Subsequently, a second ubiquitin is attached to a lysine residue of the first ubiquitin, a third ubiquitin is attached to a lysine residue of the second ubiquitin, and so on, until a chain consisting of four ubiquitin monomers is attached to the target protein (Figure 1). The ubiquitinated protein is then sent to the proteosome where it is degraded into single amino acids. In the proteosome, threonine proteases cleave solvent-exposed peptide bonds using a threonine active site residue. A representative cleavage of a diglycine peptide at pH 7 is shown in Figure 2.

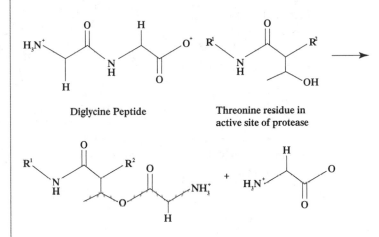

Figure 2 Threonine-dependent peptide hydrolysis

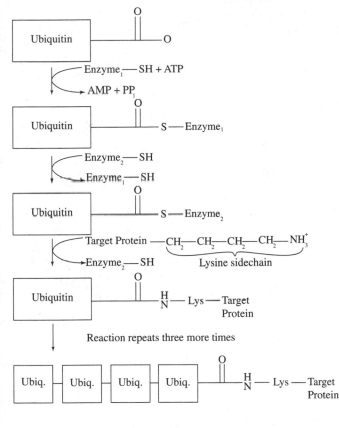

Figure 1 Ubiquitination

(Adapted from Stryer, *Biochemistry,* 3rd edition)

1. The amide bond between ubiquitin and its target protein is formed between the side chain of a lysine residue and the:

A) C-terminus of glycine 76.
B) N-terminus of glycine 76.
C) side chain of glycine 76.
D) α–carbon of glycine 76.

2. In Step 2 of ubiquitination, the ubiquitin is transferred from Enzyme$_1$ to Enzyme$_2$. This reaction is most accurately described as:

A) nucleophilic substitution.
B) transesterification.
C) trans(thio)esterification.
D) nucleophilic addition.

3. In the absence of ATP, the ubiquitination reaction would:

A) occur more slowly than in the presence of ATP.
B) occur more quickly than in the presence of ATP.
C) not be affected.
D) not occur.

4. In the threonine-dependent hydrolysis of proteins, the primary function of the threonine residue is to act as a(n):

A) acid.
B) base.
C) nucleophile.
D) electrophile.

5. Which of the following techniques would be most effective in separating lysine from a mixture of lysine, glycine, and threonine in aqueous buffer at pH 7?

A) Extraction
B) Gel electrophoresis
C) Column chromatography
D) Distillation

SOLUTIONS TO CHAPTER 7 FREESTANDING PRACTICE QUESTIONS

1. **B** Because the peptide bond is delocalized, the C—N bond has double-bond character and is difficult to break. Choice A can be eliminated because steric hindrance describes the electron density surrounding an atom, not the density associated with bonds. Choice C can be eliminated because the folding of a peptide within a protein does not affect bond strength. Choice D can be eliminated because proteins are susceptible to hydrolysis from enzymes.

2. **A** Choice A is the best because it directly addresses the energetics of ATP hydrolysis. Choice B discusses the reactivity of the released phosphate ion and not the structure of ATP itself, so it can be eliminated. Choice C can be eliminated because it describes the rate of cellular processes not the energy of ATP. Choice D can be eliminated because the structure of adenine is not related to why ATP is a good energy storage molecule.

3. **D** The secondary structure of proteins is the initial folding of the polypeptide chain into α-helices or β-pleated sheets. Choice A describes the formation of a quaternary protein, choice B can be eliminated because it describes the primary protein structure, and choice C can be eliminated because it describes the tertiary protein structure.

4. **B** Two points to consider in the melting point of fatty acids are 1) molecular weight, and 2) branching. Choices A and B both consist of eight carbons, while choices C and D each have six. Thus, it is likely that choice A or B will be the better choice based on molecular weight. Since choice A is branched and choice B is not, choice A has the lower melting point. Although all four structures may be drawn to answer this question, it is not necessary. The carbons can be counted based on the names (2 *methyl* = 2 carbons + *hexan* = 6 carbons or *but* = 4 carbons), and the methyl substituents are indicative of branching in choices A and C.

5. **C** The interconversion between α and β anomers of the same sugar is known as mutarotation. Although the mechanism of mutarotation involves both elimination, then nucleophilic addition, individually each of these two answers is incomplete (eliminate choices B and D). Tautomerism describes the equilibration between structural isomers (eliminate choice A), not anomers, which are stereoisomers.

6. **C** This problem can be approached as a two-by-two. First, consider that when aspartic acid and glutamic acid are deprotonated, they go from having neutral side chains to having a negative charge. Repulsion between these two negative charges creates an unfavorable ionic interaction (eliminate choices A and B). If the side chain of glutamic acid has a higher observed pK_a, the repulsion can be avoided somewhat since the group will be deprotonated only at higher pH, and therefore a narrower range of conditions (eliminate choice D).

7. **A** Since the peptide bond has partial double bond character, it cannot freely rotate. The peptide bond is labeled as ω, making choice A the correct answer. The rest of the labeled dihedral angles are all single bonds, and therefore can freely rotate.

SOLUTIONS TO CHAPTER 7 PRACTICE PASSAGE

1. **A** Since proteins are written from N-terminus to C-terminus, glycine 76 is the C-terminal residue with the free carbonyl shown (eliminate choice B). Glycine does not have a side chain (its R group attached to the α-carbon is a single H) so choice C can be eliminated. The α-carbon of an amino acid is next to the carbonyl, not the carbonyl carbon itself, so choice D can be eliminated.

2. **C** At the beginning of Step 2, the ubiquitin is linked to Enzyme$_1$ through a thioester bond, not a simple ester, due to the presence of sulfur in the molecule. At the end of the reaction it emerges linked to Enzyme$_2$ through a new thioester bond. Transesterification and trans(thio)esterification involve the exchange of one alcohol or thiol group, respectively, on one ester compound for another. Therefore, this reaction is best described as a trans(thio)esterification (eliminate choice B). Substitution is a tempting answer since one enzyme has been replaced by another, maintaining the same number of sigma bonds from reactant to product. However, since the interconversion of carboxylic acid derivatives occurs through an addition-elimination mechanism, choice C is a more specific answer, and choice A can be eliminated. Choice D can be eliminated since it only describes part of the mechanism.

3. **D** ATP coupling is used to drive thermodynamically unfavorable reactions that would otherwise be nonspontaneous. Therefore, in the absence of ATP this reaction would not occur. Choices A and B imply that the kinetics of the reaction would change, not the thermodynamics, and can therefore be eliminated.

4. **C** The hydroxyl group on the threonine side chain carries two lone pairs and can act as a nucleophile. Reaction 2 shows that this hydroxyl group attacks the electrophilic carbonyl carbon of the peptide bond, further implicating threonine as a nucleophile. While there is some proton transfer in this reaction, the main function of threonine is not to act as an acid or base (eliminate choices A and B), but to cause the cleavage of the peptide bond via nucleophilic addition-elimination.

5. **B** The major physical difference between lysine and the other two amino acids at pH 7 is that lysine carries an overall positive charge, as shown in Figures 1 (lysine side chain) and 2 (threonine and glycine). Gel electrophoresis separates molecules with different charges, and therefore would be the best choice for the separation. Extraction would not be effective since all of the species are charged and soluble in aqueous solution at pH 7 (eliminate choice A). Silica gel is a polar substance that would strongly attract all of the amino acids, therefore it would be very difficult to separate them using silica-based chromatography (eliminate choice C). The high molecular weight of the amino acids and ionic interactions between them will cause them to have a high vaporization point, making them nearly impossible to distill (eliminate choice D).

Organic Chemistry Glossary

After each entry, the section number in *MCAT Organic Chemistry Review* where the term is discussed is given.

1,3-diaxial interaction
A destabilizing interaction between substituents that occupy axial positions on the same side of a cyclohexane ring. [Section 4.2]

achiral
A molecule that is superimposable on its mirror image. [Section 4.2]

aldehyde
A functional group where a carbonyl is attached to one carbon group and one hydrogen. [Section 6.2]

aldol condensation
A reaction in which the enolate anion of one carbonyl reacts with the carbonyl of another compound. [Section 6.2]

alkanes
Saturated hydrocarbons of the form C_nH_{2n+2}. [Section 3.3]

amphipathic
A molecule that is both hydrophilic and hydrophobic. [Section 6.3]

anomeric center
The orientation at the anomeric center distinguishes anomers from one another. [Section 4.2]

anomers
Epimers formed by ring closure. [Section 4.2]

anti conformation
A conformation in which the two largest groups are 180° apart. [Section 4.2]

axial
A substituent orientation on rings where the group is pointed up or down, perpendicular to the plane of the ring. [Section 4.2]

Benedict's test
A test to detect aldehydes, ketones, and hemiacetals in sugars. [Section 7.3]

boiling point
The temperature at which a compound changes from a liquid into a gas. [Section 5.1]

Cahn-Ingold-Prelog rules
A set of rules for assigning absolute configuration to a stereocenter. [Section 4.2]

carbanions
Negatively charged species with a negative formal charge on carbon. [Section 4.2]

carbocations or carbonium ions
Positively charged species with a positive formal charge on carbon. [Section 4.2]

carbohydrate
A chain of hydrated carbon atoms with the molecular formula $C_nH_{2n}O_n$. [Section 7.3]

chair conformation
The most stable conformation of cyclohexane. [Section 4.2]

chemical shift
The location of a resonance in a NMR spectrum. [Section 5.2]

chiral
A molecule that cannot be superimposed on its mirror image is chiral. Most frequently this refers to an sp^3 hybridized carbon with four different groups attached to it. [Section 4.2]

cis
Substituents on the same side of a double bond or ring. [Section 4.2]

conformational isomers
Any compounds that have the same molecular formula and the same connectivity but that differ from one another by rotation about a σ bond. [Section 4.2]

ORGANIC CHEMISTRY GLOSSARY

constitutional isomers
Any compounds with the same molecular formula but whose atoms have different connectivity. [**Section 4.2**]

degree of unsaturation
A degree of unsaturation is either one ring or one π bond in a molecule. The degree of unsaturation can be calculated using the formula $[(2n + 2) - x]/2$, where n is the number of carbon atoms and x is the number of hydrogen atoms. [**Section 4.1**]

delocalized
Electron density that is spread over multiple atoms is said to be delocalized. [**Section 4.1**]

diastereomers
Stereoisomers that are not enantiomers. [**Section 4.2**]

disaccharide
Two monosaccharides bonded together. [**Section 7.3**]

distillation
A purification method based on a difference in boiling points. [**Section 5.1**]

disulfide bonds
A sulfur-sulfur bond between two cysteines that stabilizes protein structure. [**Section 7.2**]

(*E*)-alkenes
Alkenes where the two higher priority groups are on the opposite side of the double bond. [**Section 4.2**]

electron-donating groups
Groups that push (donate) electron density towards another functional group through σ or π bonds. [**Section 4.2**]

electron-withdrawing groups
Groups that pull (withdraw) electron density towards themseleves through σ or π bonds. [**Section 4.2**]

electrophiles
Electrophiles ("electron loving") are electron-deficient and typically react with nucleophiles by accepting electrons. [**Section 4.1**]

enantiomers
Molecules that are mirror images and non-superimposable. [**Section 4.2**]

enolate ion
A resonance-stabilized anion resulting from the deprotonation of a carbon atom adjacent to a carbonyl functional group. [**Section 6.2**]

epimeric center
The stereocenter at which the configuration differs in epimers. [**Section 4.2**]

epimers
Diastereomers that differ in configuration at only one of many chiral centers. [**Section 4.2**]

equatorial
A substituent orientation on rings where the group is pointed away from the center of the ring. [**Section 4.2**]

extraction
A separation technique that relies on relative solubilities of the two solvents used. [**Section 5.1**]

gas chromatography
A method that separates compounds based on their volatilities. [**Section 5.1**]

***gauche* conformation**
A conformation in which the two largest groups are 60° apart when viewed in a Newman projection. [**Section 4.2**]

geometric isomers
Diastereomers that differ in orientation of substituents around a ring or double bond. [**Section 4.2**]

glycosidic linkage
The bond between two saccharides. [**Section 7.3**]

half-chair conformation
The high-energy intermediate conformation of cyclohexane as it converts from one chair conformation into the other. [Section 4.2]

hybrid orbitals
Hybrid orbitals are a mathematical combination of atomic orbitals centered on the same atom. The total number of orbitals is conserved in their formation (i.e., the number of atomic orbitals equals the number of hybrid orbitals). [Section 4.1]

hydrophilic
Literally "water loving." [Section 7.4]

hydrophobic
Literally "water fearing." [Section 7.4]

imine formation
A reaction between an aldehyde or ketone and a primary amine to form an imine. [Section 6.2]

inductive effect
The sharing of electrons through σ bonds. [Section 4.2]

infrared spectroscopy
A method that detects the vibrations of covalent bonds and can differentiate their frequencies, which is related to the type of bond. [Section 5.2]

isomers
Any compounds that have the same molecular formula. [Section 4.2]

ketone
A functional group in which a carbonyl is attached to two carbon groups. [Section 6.2]

lipase
Enzymes that hydrolyze fats. [Section 7.4]

lipids
Oily or fatty substances that are part of cellular membranes (phospholipids), can store energy as triglycerides (in adipose cells), and can serve as the building block for steroid hormones (cholesterol). [Section 7.4]

lipid bilayer
A double layer of lipids where the polar groups line the outside and the non-polar tails compose the inside. [Section 7.4]

localized
Electrons that are confined to one orbital, either a bonding orbital or a lone-pair orbital. [Section 4.1]

melting point
The temperature at which a compound changes from a solid into a gas. [Section 5.1]

meso
A molecule that contains chiral centers and an internal plane of symmetry. [Section 4.2]

monosaccharide
Literally a "single sweet unit", also known as a simple sugar (e.g., fructose, glucose, etc.). [Section 7.3]

mutarotation
Interconversion between anomers. [Section 7.3]

nucleophile
Nucleophiles ("nucleus loving") have an unshared pair of electrons or a π bond and react with electrophiles by donating these electrons. [Section 4.1]

nucleotides
The building blocks of nucleic acids. [Section 7.5]

oligosaccharide
Several monosaccharides bonded together. [Section 7.3]

ORGANIC CHEMISTRY GLOSSARY

optically active
Compounds that rotate the plane of polarized light are optically active. A pair of enantiomers will rotate the plane of polarized light in equal, but opposite directions. [Section 4.2]

peptide bond
The bond that links amino acids together formed between the carboxyl group of one amino acid and the amino group of another. [Section 7.2]

pi (π) bonds
A π bond consists of two electrons localized above and below a nodal plane; π bonds are formed from overlap of two unhybridized p orbitals on adjacent atoms. [Section 4.1]

polysaccharide
Many monosaccharides bonded together. [Section 7.3]

protease
A protein enzyme that performs proteolysis. [Section 7.2]

proteolysis
Hydrolysis of a protein by another protein. [Section 7.2]

racemic mixture
An equal mixture of two enantiomers is said to be racemic; racemic mixtures do not rotate the plane of polarized light because one enantiomer cancels out the rotation of the other. [Section 4.2]

resonance
The sharing of electrons through π bonds. [Section 4.2]

ring strain
Instability due to deviation of bond angles from optimal geometry. [Section 4.2]

saponification
The hydrolysis of esters by treatment with a basic solution. [Section 6.3]

saturated
A molecule is saturated if it contains no π bonds and no rings. [Section 4.1]

sigma (σ) bonds
A σ bond consists of two electrons localized between two nuclei; σ bonds are formed by overlap of two hybridized orbitals. [Section 4.1]

stereoisomers
Any compounds with the same molecular formula and connectivity that differ only in the spatial arrangement of atoms, are known as stereoisomers. Note that if the compounds only differ by rotation around a sigma bond they are not stereoisomers but *conformational* isomers. [Section 4.2]

tautomers
Readily interconvertible constitutional isomers. [Section 6.2]

thin-layer chromatography (TLC)
A rapid technique used to separate compounds based on their polarity. [Section 5.1]

trans
Substituents on opposite sides of a double bond. [Section 4.2]

twist boat conformation
The local energy minimum for cyclohexane as it converts from one chair conformation to the other. [Section 4.2]

unsaturated
A molecule is unsaturated if it contains at least one π bond or ring. [Section 4.1]

van der Waals forces
A general term for intermolecular forces, often used to describe London dispersion forces: forces between temporary dipoles formed in nonpolar molecules formed because of a temporary asymmetric electron distribution. [Section 5.1]

wavenumber
The reciprocal of wavelength, expressed in reciprocal centimeters (cm^{-1}). [**Section 5.2**]

(*Z*)-alkenes
Alkenes where the two high priority groups are on the same side of the double bond. [**Section 4.2**]

zwitterion
A molecule with both positive and negative formal charges. [**Section 7.1**]

Summary of Reactions

Oxidation of Alcohols

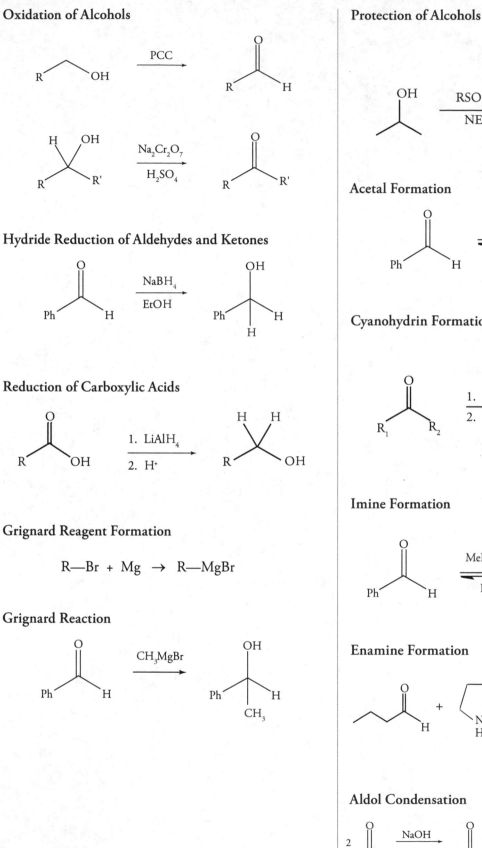

Hydride Reduction of Aldehydes and Ketones

Reduction of Carboxylic Acids

Grignard Reagent Formation

$$R—Br + Mg \rightarrow R—MgBr$$

Grignard Reaction

Protection of Alcohols

Acetal Formation

Cyanohydrin Formation

Imine Formation

Enamine Formation

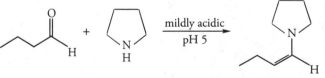

Aldol Condensation

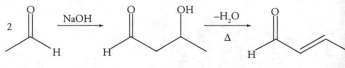

SUMMARY OF REACTIONS

Decarboxylation

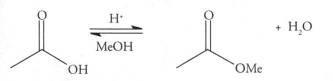

Esterification

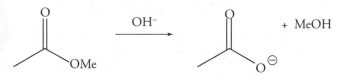

Saponification

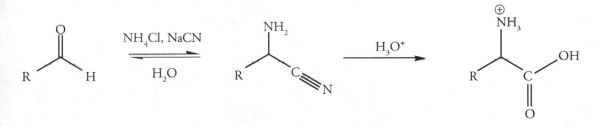

Unimolecular Substitution (S_N1)

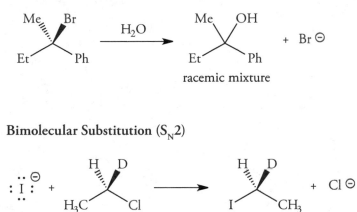

Bimolecular Substitution (S_N2)

Strecker Synthesis of Amino Acids

Gabriel Malonic Ester Synthesis of Amino Acids

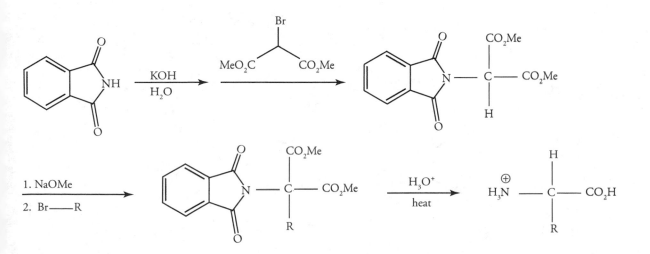

Organic Chemistry
Appendix

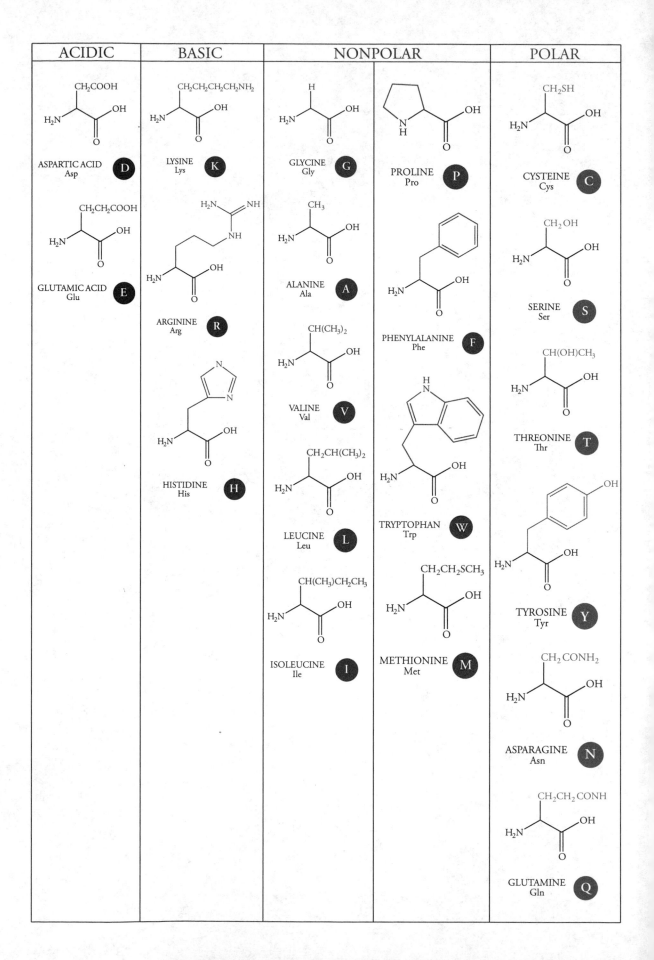

ACIDIC	BASIC	NONPOLAR		POLAR

ACIDIC

ASPARTIC ACID Asp — D
CH₂COOH

GLUTAMIC ACID Glu — E
CH₂CH₂COOH

BASIC

LYSINE Lys — K
CH₂CH₂CH₂CH₂NH₂

ARGININE Arg — R

HISTIDINE His — H

NONPOLAR

GLYCINE Gly — G

ALANINE Ala — A
CH₃

VALINE Val — V
CH(CH₃)₂

LEUCINE Leu — L
CH₂CH(CH₃)₂

ISOLEUCINE Ile — I
CH(CH₃)CH₂CH₃

PROLINE Pro — P

PHENYLALANINE Phe — F

TRYPTOPHAN Trp — W

METHIONINE Met — M
CH₂CH₂SCH₃

POLAR

CYSTEINE Cys — C
CH₂SH

SERINE Ser — S
CH₂OH

THREONINE Thr — T
CH(OH)CH₃

TYROSINE Tyr — Y

ASPARAGINE Asn — N
CH₂CONH₂

GLUTAMINE Gln — Q
CH₂CH₂CONH